Intuitive Acupuncture

Intuitive Acupuncture

JOHN HAMWEE

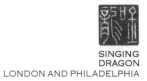

SINGING
DRAGON
LONDON AND PHILADELPHIA

First published in 2016
by Singing Dragon
an imprint of Jessica Kingsley Publishers
73 Collier Street
London N1 9BE, UK
and
400 Market Street, Suite 400
Philadelphia, PA 19106, USA

www.singingdragon.com

Library of Congress Cataloging in Publication Data
Hamwee, John, author.
 Intuitive acupuncture / John Hamwee.
   p. ; cm.
 Includes bibliographical references.
 ISBN 978-1-84819-273-7 (alk. paper)
 I. Title.
 [DNLM: 1. Acupuncture. 2. Intuition. WB 369]
 RM184
 615.8'92--dc23
                    2015021616

British Library Cataloguing in Publication Data
A CIP catalogue record for this book is available from the British Library

ISBN 978 1 84819 273 7
eISBN 978 0 85701 220 3

Printed and bound in the United States

For Cathy

Acknowledgements

My first debt is to my teachers: Meriel Darby, Angie and John Hicks and Dr Fritz Smith.

I am grateful to those who, by generously sharing their wisdom and experience, have made it a much better book than I could have written on my own: Myra Connell, Jenny Craig, Sophie Mitchell, Frances Turner, James Unsworth and Allegra Wint.

Jessica Kingsley has been a wonderful publisher and I could not have written this without her support, encouragement and expertise.

And finally my thanks go to all my patients who have allowed me to practise on them and learn from each treatment.

Contents

Preface

This is not a 'how to do it' book, still less a 'how you ought to do it' book. My aim is to help you become more aware of your own innate skills and to appreciate some of the things you already do in the treatment room, though perhaps without fully realising what they are and how valuable they can be. I hope too that it will increase your sensitivity to those skills so that you can use them more often and with more confidence; partly because there is satisfaction in that, but also because I think it will enable you to meet the needs of your patients with more accuracy and clarity.

A colleague I much admire and respect, a more experienced practitioner than me, commented on an earlier book I'd written that she really liked the quotes. I almost took offence. I almost heard her say that the only parts of the book she liked were precisely the ones I hadn't written. But then I saw the value in what she was saying. In the course of my reading I had come across wonderful ideas, remarkable perceptions, flashes of brilliance by writers with deep wisdom and a command of language. Why wouldn't I want to use their words instead of mine? That's why you'll find so many quotes in this book. Here is the first, by Ted Kaptchuk:

> Stephanus, a sixth century Greek doctor...said that medicine suffers from a fundamental contradiction; its theory grasps universals while its practice deals with individuals. (Kaptchuk 1989, p.104)

As we struggle to find the right diagnosis or to understand why a treatment seems not to be working as it should, it is a comfort to realise that we are indeed on the horns of a dilemma, and an inescapable one at that. Most of the time we just live with it and manage to get by. But one of the gifts of intuition is that it can swerve us past those horns. In a moment of insight you can suddenly arrive at a diagnosis that is in all the books and also fits the unique patient in front of you perfectly; or you craft a highly individualised treatment for an unusual condition and later realise that what you have done is an exemplar of something described in the Nei Jing.

And just in case you suspect that intuition is something only for rather weird or way-out practitioners, here is what one genius, J.M. Keynes, said of another. Writing of Sir Isaac Newton, perhaps the most famous scientist of them all, he commented, 'I fancy his pre-eminence is due to his muscles of intuition being the strongest and most enduring with which a man had ever been gifted' (Keynes, cited in Myers 2002, p.61).

CHAPTER 1

Intuition

Thirty years ago a woman sat at her kitchen table. She looked up and saw a man she didn't know walking past the window. She said to herself, I'm going to marry him. She did, and they have been married ever since.

A well-known novelist recently spoke of a similar experience. 'I walked up a field I'd not walked up before and over the brow of the field there appeared the ridge line of a house, and by the time I'd reached the house, and I can't explain this, I knew it was the only place I could possibly live' (Garner 2014). And he has lived there for over fifty years.

Perhaps the reason these examples are so striking is simply because the predictions came true; maybe we all have what we think of as astonishing insights, but the overwhelming majority of them turn out to be wrong and so are forgotten. Even so, there is something compelling about these stories. They seem to open a window onto a truth that we don't normally encounter in our everyday thoughts and plans.

Experiences like these are highly valued in a number of Eastern traditions and whole disciplines have been developed to foster them. A well-known example comes from the practice of Zen Buddhism, where the student is instructed to ponder such imponderables as the look of her face before she was born or the sound of one hand clapping. There is no possibility of finding an

answer through the normal processes of thought and enquiry
– which is, of course, the whole point. 'Sartori [Japanese for
awakening] really designates the sudden and intuitive way of
seeing into anything...one seeks and seeks but cannot find. One
then gives up and the answer comes by itself' (Watts 1962, p.181).

If not exactly fostered by conventional medical practice and
procedures, there is at least a recognition that the times when
'the answer comes by itself' are both common and valid. 'The
best [doctors] seem to have sixth sense about disease. They feel
its presence, know it to be there, perceive its gravity before any
intellectual process can define, catalog, and put it into words'
(LaCombe, cited in Mukherjee 2011, p.128).

There are many medical stories about what this author calls
a sixth sense; here is one:

> That night the nurse couldn't stay away from the patient's
> room, even though she was assigned to someone else's
> care... She found him 'sort of pale and anxious', and even
> though he was still conscious she called the doctors and,
> sure enough, just as the doctors arrived the patient began to
> die... The pulmonary embolism was caught, and the patient
> was saved. In trying to explain her need to check on the
> patient, the nurse could only say, 'I had a suspicion there
> was something wrong with him.' (Schultz 1999, p.43)

A neurosurgeon points out that intuition is inescapable,
however scientific the system of medicine:

> Consider headache for a moment. This very common
> symptom may be the result of eye strain; meningitis (many
> different infectious agents); hemorrhage (from several
> dozen causes); increased intracranial pressure (from many
> different types of tumor...a head injury with bleeding; a
> blood clot, failure to absorb fluid, excess production of
> fluid); vascular irritation (dilated blood vessels such as
> in migraine); or muscle tension – among others! ...most

thinking physicians are aware that, ultimately, it is their intuition which allows them to 'guess' which tests to order in order to make a 'suspected' diagnosis. (Shealey and Myss 1988, pp.61–2)

When practitioners, whether of Western or Eastern medicine, reflect on what they actually do, as opposed to what they were taught to do, they often comment on this combination of a subjective guess and an objective assessment.

I decided to start my treatment by taking advantage of Manaka's yin-yang channel balancing model... I did this by treating the Liver-Small Intestine polar channel pair on the first visit. My thought process at this time was a blur of intuitive insight and rational logic. (Birch 1997, p.132)

I am sure that many diagnoses are the product of this kind of blur. Recently I was treating a young woman who, although she seemed well in general, had not had a period for more than six years. As it was the fourth or fifth session I was beginning to become confident of my diagnosis and I had enough feedback from previous treatments to have some idea of what was good for her. I bent over her ankle to needle Ki 3, but for some reason it didn't feel right. I stepped back, a bit puzzled. Then I wondered if Ki 6 would be better. I felt that point too, but as I was doing so I felt drawn instead to Ki 5. I knew this was the Xi Cleft point, but that was about all; I have hardly ever used it. So I went and looked it up in *A Manual of Acupuncture* and the very first indication for that point is amenorrhoea. I think it is true to say that logic got me to the Kidney channel, but intuition took me to Ki 5.

This is one way intuition can work, which is by giving a tiny hint as to how best to proceed or a mere glimpse of some possibility or a fleeting impression of a quality of energy. It might arrive as a half-heard voice in your ear or as a nudge that pushes you ever so gently off the familiar path.

We tend to think of reasoning as primary and intuition as secondary, but it is probably more accurate to see them as equal and complementary.

> The manner in which the mathematician works his way towards discovery, by shifting his confidence from intuition to computation and back again from computation to intuition, while never releasing his hold on either of the two, represents in miniature...the reasoning powers of man. (Polanyi 1958, p.131)

And here is the man who created the polio vaccine, reflecting on his scientific career: 'Only by cultivating and refining the processes of intuition and reason complementarily, only by reconciling each in the service of the other, can we achieve the wisdom we seek' (Salk 1983, p.18).

All professions use this combination of the two kinds of thinking. My father was a lawyer and good at the relentless logic of following an argument. But what he was really good at was knowing whether or not a case could be won; some of them that looked easy he refused to take on; others that seemed hopeless he threw himself into with confidence and came out triumphant. I am sure he could point to various features of these cases that suggested success in spite of the odds, just as an experienced acupuncturist faced with a very ill patient can spot energetic imbalances, which, if treated, should lead the patient back to health. In both instances, experience has shown them something that others might not have noticed; maybe something they didn't even consciously notice themselves. Or perhaps it's not so much that experienced practitioners see something that others miss, more that they place a great deal of weight on some particular sign or symptom that others might regard as unimportant. Certainly my father would have said he had hunches, and thought no more about it.

An example from my own practice is a young man with a long history of bowel problems. He had seen many specialists and taken many kinds of medication, but still had a dozen or more bowel movements a day, and most of them were urgent. With a chronic condition like this I don't usually know if I can help until I have seen the patient a few times, until I have mulled over, refined or changed my diagnosis and until I have found out which treatments seem to bring about an improvement and which do not. But within seconds of the first needles being inserted at the very first session this young man started to laugh. And it was one of those bubbling laughs that comes up irresistibly from the very depths of a person's being. He tried to control it, but it broke out again. He apologised; I assured him it was alright. It stopped, then started again. I couldn't help smiling. He shed a few tears too, which were quickly wiped away. In all, I suppose it lasted for about five minutes. After that I was practically certain he would get better. You could say that the response from his body and mind was so instinctive and so unequivocal that I gave more weight to it than to all the history of his intractable problems and failed remedies, but actually it didn't seem like that at the time. I just knew, and there was nothing much more to say about it.

If you reach a conclusion by logical deduction then, even if you did it in an instant, you can retrace the steps and work out how you got there. That means, for instance, that you and others can check to see if there are any flaws in your reasoning. In one of the colleges where I was trained we were encouraged to decide how to treat a patient by drawing a diagram on which the main signs and symptoms were connected by arrows to the diagnosis, which in turn led to treatment principles, which then suggested specific points to be needled. As a process it helps the acupuncturist to ponder causation, to organise thoughts and to become aware of any inconsistencies in reasoning. With intuitive thinking, by contrast, we don't know how we know something, we just do. The notion arrives unbidden. It may make sense and it may not, but the experience is less like thinking and more like having a drink when you're thirsty – instinctive, natural and with a sense of rightness about it.

Rationality and logical thinking are both taught explicitly and implicitly in schools and universities in the West. But in spite of the fact that all the eminent thinkers and scientists I have quoted regard intuition as equally important, there are no courses in it and hardly anyone has researched it. You get hunches or you don't, seems to be the attitude. Some of them are useful; most of them are not. The good ones and the poor ones appear to come equally randomly, so what is there to study? How can intuition be taught as a skill, or improved if you already have it? Fortunately, a few people have applied themselves to these questions, and relating their work to the practice of acupuncture sheds much light on what we do – and could do better.

Intuition as recognition

Herbert Simon, a Nobel Prize winner, put forward the following concise description and explanation of intuition:

> In everyday speech, we use the word intuition to describe a problem-solving or question-answering performance that is speedy and for which the expert is unable to describe in detail the reasoning or other process that produced the answer. The situation has provided a cue; this cue has given the expert access to information stored in memory, and the

information provides the answer. Intuition is nothing more and nothing less than recognition. (Simon 1992, p.155)

In other words, there is nothing magical at all about intuition. Experts can't explain how intuitions appear in consciousness simply because they aren't aware of how much they know, nor can they track the lightning speed with which they compare the present case to the ones 'stored in memory' in order to find a fit. But that is what they are doing and that is all they are doing. The intuition arrives at the moment when a good comparison is made. The quotation continues with this example: 'A large part of the chess master's expertise lies in his or her intuitive (recognition) capabilities based, in turn, on large amounts of stored and indexed knowledge derived from training and experience' (Simon 1992, p.155).

All of this applies directly to the process of acupuncture diagnosis. The practitioner notices a sign, hears about the symptoms and is instantly riffling through the well-known syndromes, phases or elements in her head until that moment when she realises that what she is seeing is Spleen Qi deficiency combined with Heart Blood deficiency, for example, or an Earth constitutional type with Fire as a sub-type. Quite complex diagnoses, but then the expert remembers having seen these things many times before and recognises this patient as fundamentally the same as the others she has seen with that same combination. As I shall have a good deal more to say about this kind of intuition I am going to call it 'unconscious inference'.

Here is an example. When a new patient walked into my treatment room recently I was immediately struck by her pale face, dry hair and the lassitude with which she looked around, put her bags down slowly and settled herself in a chair. Then she told me that she kept forgetting things and didn't sleep well – all signs and symptoms of Blood deficiency, pretty much a textbook case actually. I might have looked no further, but there were a few things that gave me pause for thought. I looked at her tongue and it wasn't pale; on the contrary it had a vibrant colour and a healthy moss. Then I discovered that her periods were absolutely regular, pain free and with a moderate flow of red blood for three days. And once I started to talk to her about her life I discovered that she held down a demanding job and didn't find it exhausting; on the contrary, she told me she loved working late when everyone else had gone home.

When signs and symptoms are contradictory or inconsistent – and I am tempted to ask, when are they not? – I usually just struggle on trying to make sense of things. Sometimes I decide to ignore the difficulty and focus on one aspect of the patient's energy and see what happens when I treat it. But occasionally I get lucky and suddenly understand. It wasn't so much that this woman was Blood deficient, I realised one day, as that her Fire had gone out. A pretty obvious alternative once I'd thought of it. And if Herbert Simon had been there no doubt he would have nodded his head and commented that I had picked up some cue, perhaps a lack of laughter in her voice or an evident lack of joy in her life, and that had triggered memories of patients I have treated in the past using mainly Fire channels and Fire points, and I recognised her as essentially the same. That's exactly what intuition does, he would say, and there's no mystery to it at all.

It is really helpful to have this concept of unconscious inference. For one thing, it acts as a caution to inexperienced practitioners. Until they have seen many patients they would do well, according to this view, to be very wary of any intuitive diagnosis; they simply don't have a sufficient memory bank to identify a new patient as like a host of others who have been successfully diagnosed and treated in the past. And it also suggests that when an experienced practitioner has a hunch and suddenly wants to do points based on an unlikely and unexpected diagnosis, there is a way of checking before taking action. A question like 'Who does this patient remind me of?' might bring the unconscious recognition up to consciousness; and then it can be examined to see if it really is accurate. Another possibility is to ask, 'What is it about this patient that makes me reject the obvious diagnosis?' Again, this question nudges the practitioner to make explicit what has been an instinctive reaction and response, and then it can be examined and tested.

And this ability to check up on a sudden idea means that a practitioner can learn to use her intuition better. If each time she does a treatment based on this kind of diagnosis she makes a note that she has done so, then when she sees that patient again she can find out if her idea was accurate or not. And if she keeps this up over the course of a few months she can then look back over a range of instances and see how reliable her intuition really is. And there is more information available too; when I did this myself I found that my intuition was pretty accurate when I was treating muscular-skeletal conditions and acute conditions generally, much less so when I was treating patients with chronic conditions. And finding out why that was so taught me quite a bit about my strengths and weaknesses as a practitioner.

Beyond recognition

Michael Polanyi, a chemist and philosopher of science, has put flesh onto the bare bones of intuition as recognition. The best way to appreciate the essence of his ideas is to answer the following question quickly and without pausing to think. Imagine you are riding a bicycle and it starts to topple to the left. Which way do you turn the handlebars?

You might have found it quite hard to answer the question. You might even have got the answer wrong (as did a close friend who is a keen cyclist; in fact you steer to the left). All of which is very odd because when you are riding a bicycle you know the answer without having to think about it, and you never get it wrong. Polanyi's explanation is that we all have what he calls tacit knowledge. That is, we know a lot of things without being at all aware that we know them. He often uses the example of recognising a friend's face in a crowd. The recognition is instant and unmistakable, but it is really difficult to say exactly what it is that makes us so sure. We might try listing the colour of his hair, the shape of his skull and so on, but what is actually happening is not the same as a kind of totting up of all his individual features.

These are homely examples, but he doesn't see tacit knowledge as simply a kind of useful addition to our explicit knowledge, helpful in normal everyday life. In summarising his argument he points out that the most rigorous of rational thinking actually depends on tacit knowledge:

> Hademard says that he used to make more mistakes in calculation than his own pupils, but that he more quickly discovered them because the result did not *look* right... Gauss is widely quoted as having said: 'I have had my solutions for a long time but I did not yet know how I am to arrive at them.' (Polanyi 1958, pp.130–1, italics in original)

In other words, behind and beyond the logic and the calculations lies an enormous amount of tacit knowledge. This applies directly to the practice of acupuncture. Here are two examples – I am sure you can easily think of your own – from patients I saw on the day I wrote this.

A woman, in her late fifties, a new patient, talked to me for about half an hour, telling me that her main complaints were recurrent back pain and occasional migraines. She explained some of her medical history and recounted a little bit about her life. At one point she told me that she had wet her bed as a child and her father called her 'pisser'. Was this an absolutely crucial piece of information or not? Sometimes, of course, it is easy to decide because the background information relates directly to the symptoms, but often, as here, it does not. She also told me that she had been quite promiscuous as a young woman; again, was this important or not? In deciding what to write down, what to remember, I was constantly making decisions of this kind. Although I had no way of knowing for sure, I wrote down all the details of the first and ignored the second. Even now, having had time to reflect on it, I would be hard put to explain why. In short, all the way through the conversation I was using tacit knowledge to select information that was going to help me reach a diagnosis and choose a treatment.

Another patient, a woman nearing menopause, told me that she sweats a lot in bed at night, and indeed her pulses always speak of Yin deficiency. At the same time she says she has had a cold, which in mid-June was so bad that she had to delay her holiday until it was over. Then she adds that a large boil has come up recently on her back and is now weeping puss. I looked at the boil and her tongue and decided – nothing clever about this – that I would need to clear Phlegm first and then treat Kidney Yin deficiency.

I could have just gone ahead and done it, but something made me ask more about her being hot in bed at night. Did she throw off the covers and then get cold and then have to put them back on again? She looked surprised. 'Oh no, not at all,' she said. She had to sleep with a heavy duvet (this is in June) and what's more it had to be doubled over on her feet. I asked her why and she replied, 'Because otherwise I can't feel my body.'

Extraordinary, isn't it, how patients tell you the strangest things as if they were perfectly normal? But what I'm getting at here is the tacit knowledge that made me ask more about her feeling hot in bed. After all, given that she is Yin deficient, it was what I would have expected. Mulling it over, I still can't put my finger on what it was that made me pursue the point, but the following, at least, are involved: a practised attention; an understanding of energy in the human body and the signs of its distortion; and a set of criteria that discriminate between the crucial, the interesting and the irrelevant. And, in the moment, all of them are tacit.

It might seem that this concept of tacit knowledge simply adds to Herbert Simon's description of intuition, but in fact it points the way to a radical alternative. If we do indeed operate much of the time with tacit knowledge, then it can't be true that our intuitions are unconscious inferences that can be fully explained if only we were to take the time and trouble to do so. The whole point about tacit knowledge is that it can't be made explicit. Whatever its nature and its source, it is such a complex amalgam of memories, thoughts, emotions, experiences, half-remembered impressions and so on, some of which are entirely personal and some of which are common to the times and culture in which we live, that we don't know what's in it nor how it influences us. So to say we have retraced the steps of our decision-making as if it did not depend on tacit knowledge is a bit like pretending we have walked a path when we've simply looked at it on a map.

This is not just a theoretical issue. Ignoring tacit knowledge and believing we can explain intuition as a logical but unconscious process leads us to assume that we can know exactly what we are doing. So if, after the event and with a bit of effort, an expert's quick and intuitive diagnosis can be spelled out in the way that Herbert Simon suggests, then it can be made into an algorithm that can be put into a computer. To make a diagnosis as good as that of the expert, all a practitioner has to do is to type in the signs and symptoms and the computer will give the result. At the time of writing, algorithms like this are used in America not just by clinicians but also by insurance companies and government departments. Once a patient has such a computerised diagnosis then it doesn't merely state what treatment is to be given, it also says how long it should take and how much it should cost. The implications are enormous and they are not ones that sit well with the practice of acupuncture.

The following quotation is not about acupuncture, but it does speak to the way we work and to what we may have to defend about it:

> Who you are is quite apparent to anyone who takes the time to quiet down and allow the experience of being with you to be the focus of their attention. Similarly, you can know much more about other people than you usually notice or articulate. You can sense what someone is like by simply being with them... The quality of a person's presence can be clearly perceived by anyone who cares to tune in to their intuitive abilities. (Vaughan 1979, p.105)

By 'the quality of a person's presence' we can just as easily read the quality of a person's energy. And the idea of tuning into intuitive abilities is suggestive. Given that we all have them, how do we tune into them more often and more accurately? There must be some skills and techniques involved. The distinguished acupuncturists who wrote the following clearly think so: '...emphasis on the diagnosis of an individual's constitutional imbalance means that the practitioners must rely largely on their sensory and intuitive skills' (Hicks, Hicks and Mole 2004, p.xi). Although they are writing about one form of acupuncture diagnosis, I think it applies, at least to some extent, to them all.

Sudden knowing

When I asked a very experienced practitioner how he arrived at his diagnoses he said to me in all seriousness, 'I have no idea what I am doing.' When I pressed him, saying he must know what he was doing, he told me that he sat and listened to his patients, barely paying attention to the content of what they were saying, until he knew what to do. He went on to say that sometimes it would take a few minutes, occasionally half an hour or more, but rarely did he not have a moment of insight, a kind of sudden understanding. I believe that he must have great 'sensory and intuitive skills' even though he has not troubled to formulate them, and that he is using tacit knowledge all the time to yield the intuitions with which he works. I want to distinguish what he seems to be doing from the more usual unconscious inferences, so I am going to call his kind of intuition, 'sudden knowing'.

The two people at the start of the chapter – the woman who chose her future husband as he walked past the window and the author who knew he was going to live in a certain house the moment he first saw it – they both had these sudden knowings. What happened to them can't be explained as any kind of unconscious inference. It wasn't that these people had an idea that, if carefully traced back, made sense; it was more that they had an experience.

It is this kind of intuition that Jung must have had in mind when he wrote: 'This term [intuition] does not denote something contrary to reason, but something outside the province of reason' (Jung, cited in Vaughan 1979, p.57).

There are plenty of famous examples of sudden knowing in the arts and sciences. Andrew Wiles worked for many years, alone and in secret, trying to prove Fermat's last theorem, a problem that had defeated mathematicians for more than three centuries. I watched as he spoke on television of the moment when, after all the calculations, the dead ends and red herrings, he just knew. He couldn't believe he hadn't seen the proof before. Tears came to his eyes at the memory of it and he had to turn away from the camera, unable to carry on.

Another example comes from Fritz Smith, a medical doctor, osteopath and acupuncturist. Each of the three forms of medicine he knew and practised was based on a view of the human body that he held to be true because each led to effective treatments; but at the same time they were all completely inconsistent and incompatible. For many years he puzzled over how this could be. Then one day, as he recounted to me, 'the top of my head opened up, information poured in and I saw the relationship between anatomy, physiology and energy in the human body.'

These accounts are especially interesting as they are of people who are not only expert in their fields but who also have given sustained thought to problems that their professional colleagues had avoided, ignored or decided were insoluble. No doubt Herbert Simon would point out that these pioneers have vast amounts of 'information stored in memory', but still, what is going on cannot possibly be unconscious inference. The breakthrough, when it comes, is too radical, too far from what has been possible before. Rather than an inference there is an epiphany; rather than a thought, a vision.

Ted Kaptchuk talks about this when he discusses what he calls the three levels of the physician's art:

> This third level of artistry has to do with an intimate, intuitive and immediate encounter with humanity... I first learned about this kind of vision from Dr Hong, my first teacher... He just knew. His intuition had been refined in the crucible of experience that gave him capacities beyond

what is ordinarily thought possible. (Kaptchuk 2000, pp.288, 291)

The use of the word 'artistry' in this context points towards something that is beyond the practical and the routine. Here is another scholar and practitioner reflecting on the issue:

> The skilful exercise of the craft [of Chinese medicine], its art if you like, expresses itself in understanding illness in such a manner that there remain no doubts, no unwarranted conjectures, no ifs and maybes, no ad-hoc hypotheses. One of the expressions of such skill seems to be simplicity; the ability to select from a thousand and one herbs and acupuncture points the one or two that are right. Interestingly enough, philosophers, mathematicians, physicists and many others seem to share with Chinese physicians this sense of aesthetic efficacy. (Scheid 1997, p.59)

Heaven knows, I spend enough time in the treatment room with 'ifs and maybes', having doubts about my diagnoses and making ad-hoc hypotheses about what is going on when the pulses, or the patients, don't respond as I hope they will, so it would be wonderful to be able to work with such complete confidence. And not only for me – for I am sure that any treatment works best when there is the kind of simple clarity about it that comes from the practitioner's confidence, even if it is not technically perfect or even particularly accurate. I think that is because the treatment gives a clear direction to the patient's energy so it is more effective than a muddled instruction; or maybe it's rather that confidence acts as a placebo; or perhaps it's some combination of the two.

There is nothing rational about these sudden knowings. They flash up unimagined possibilities; they startle with sudden insight; they see in the dark and hear the unsaid. Fundamentally they are a mystery. They give remarkable powers and they have brought about profound change in the arts, in science and society as well as in medicine. In the treatment room they can yield a perception of the patient and the state of her energy that is utterly compelling. And they need to be used carefully. Paranoias, fears, anxieties, fantasies, wishful thinking, projections and megalomania can all masquerade as authentic intuitions. For this kind of intuition does not evaluate, and has no powers of judgement or discrimination. It is no good expecting it to check up on itself; it can't.

This is especially important because, according to the results of tests with the Myers-Briggs type indicator, the overwhelming majority of people who work one-to-one in a therapeutic setting are intuitive types. In other words, we acupuncturists are likely to be naturally prone to both the virtues and the vices of intuition. Jung has this to say about intuitive types:

> It goes without saying that such a type is uncommon...he can render exceptional service... Because he is able, when oriented more to people than things, to make an intuitive diagnosis of their abilities and potentialities, he can also 'make' men... He brings his vision to life, he presents it convincingly and with dramatic fire, he embodies it, so to speak. But this is not play acting, it is a kind of fate. (Jung 1971, p.369)

If this sounds familiar to you, then what follows will confirm much of what you already know, though I hope it will also help you to enhance and make the most of it. And if you don't identify with this description then here is an opportunity to learn a new skill that can bring enormous benefits to you and to your patients.

CHAPTER 2

Attention

I will always remember the first time I watched an acupuncturist at work, long before I even thought of qualifying myself. I knew absolutely nothing about what she was doing but I could see that she was working with the kind of sure-footedness that made me think of a skilled climber going up bare rock or a jazz musician improvising a riff. I was dazzled. As an academic I was used to mulling things over at great length and hesitating before I reached any conclusions, which I would then hedge about with reservations and provisos. But here was this acupuncturist making decisions on the hoof and then implementing them instantly. In fact, I wasn't even sure that there was a gap between the thought and the action.

I didn't think much more about it as I did my training, preoccupied as I was with point location, pulse taking and the rest. But soon after I qualified I had the opportunity to watch another very experienced practitioner at work and this time I could be more analytical about what I was witnessing. He asked questions that seemed to be irrelevant, but each one led the patient to reveal something important. He chose points, and remarkably few of them, that would never have occurred to me. And he got pulse changes the like of which I haven't seen since. It was a masterclass given to someone too inexperienced to really learn the lessons.

But I did come away with one abiding question: How did he know? How did he know to ask a forty-year-old man if his mother was given ether when he was born (she had been) and why did he think to ask it just as he palpated the right foot? Or, to take another example, what led him to tonify LI 11 (a point I have only ever needled with even or reducing technique) on a woman waiting, in some distress, for the outcome of tests for cancer? What's more, the point clearly touched something deep in her; the slow flood of colour into her face, the aliveness returning to her skin and the relief she expressed so poignantly afterwards gave convincing proof of that.

In order to ask the key question, or needle the key point, it seemed to me that he must have noticed something or sensed something of which I was completely unaware; or perhaps it wasn't one thing but a host of tiny things that cumulatively carried one unequivocal message. Whatever it was, I wanted to find out how he did it.

Both these practitioners had deep knowledge of the theory and long experience of their craft, but that didn't seem to me to be enough to explain the way they worked. They weren't thinking what to do, at least not in the way I understood thinking. It was partly that they were working so fast that they couldn't be reasoning their way to a conclusion; but again it was more than that. It was a bit like when you pick up the phone and hear your child's voice on the other end of the line, and even though she is saying something innocuous you know there is something wrong. Similarly, these practitioners seemed to be reaching their diagnoses instantly and intuitively; they just knew. Or, perhaps, and even more intriguingly, they just knew the patient. The questions that seemed to me miraculous simply arose from that perception. Pulses and tongue confirmed it. Point selection was a way to treat it. Needling made it happen.

Fortunately one of them gave me the key to how he did it. 'I work,' he said, 'with attention not intention.' Although that was over twenty years ago, I am still discovering more and more implications of that remarkable statement.

For one thing, in an age of mission statements, aims and objectives, goals and targets – all expressions of intention – it is a radical manifesto. Western medicine is based on intention too; drugs are developed to catalyse or inhibit highly specific chemical reactions and surgery seeks to remove the particular diseased or damaged part of the body and nothing else. To work with attention not intention is a fundamental challenge to our normal way of thinking.

At first sight, paying attention seems like a rather weak and passive activity; it reminds me of having to listen to a rather dull teacher at school. But when I recall that the classic meditation technique is to pay the closest possible attention to the breath I realise there must be more to it than that. 'Breath is the bridge which connects life to consciousness, which unites your body to your thoughts. Whenever your mind becomes scattered, use your breath as the means to take hold of your mind again' (Hanh 1976, p.15).

This is more than the ordinary attention of everyday life and it can reveal more than we normally notice. Here is an account of how it works:

> ...it occurred to me that there must be two quite different ways of perceiving. Only a tiny act of will was necessary to pass from one to the other, yet this act seemed sufficient to change the face of the world. The first way of perceiving seemed to be the automatic one, the kind of attention which my mind gave to everyday affairs when it was left to itself... The second way of perceiving seemed to occur when...there was no need to select one item to look at rather than another, so it became possible to look at the whole at once. To attend

to something yet want nothing from it, these seemed to be the essentials of the second way of perceiving... Once when ill in bed...I had found myself staring vacantly at a faded cyclamen and happened to remember to say to myself, 'I want nothing.' Immediately I was so flooded with the crimson of the petals that I thought I had never before known what colour was. (Milner 1986, p.178)

If our treatments are to be genuinely holistic then we will need to use this second way of perceiving, which makes it 'possible to look at the whole at once'. And the way to do that, according to this author, is to 'want nothing from it'.

I don't think she means to imply that we have to be indifferent to the outcome, indifferent to whether or not our patients get well; rather she is suggesting that we look at them without trying to discover anything in particular, without being tempted to analyse or apply categories, and certainly without seeking their approval or wanting them to like us. Attention with no ulterior motive is another way of putting it.

I only really understood the force of all this when I moved to another part of the country and closed down my practice. As a way of saying goodbye to it all and learning something about what I had been doing, I thought it would be useful to go through all my notes and see which patients had got better and which ones had not. Perhaps I would be able to draw some clear conclusions; maybe I didn't have much success with muscular-skeletal problems or headaches, and so would refer such patients to someone else. But there seemed to be no pattern. Some patients who were highly sceptical about acupuncture got better and others who were deeply interested in it didn't. Some with very long-standing and quite acute conditions got instant improvement and others who had minor but irritating symptoms did not. I couldn't find any criteria that discriminated accurately between the two groups.

Until, that is, I had the notion of shifting my attention from the patients to myself. Then I discovered that there were indeed two groups who tended not to do well. The first consisted of people about whom I was especially anxious that treatment would work for them: a young woman wanting to start a family but whose periods had unaccountably stopped; a very good artist with early onset of Parkinson's disease; and an old friend who really wanted to understand why I had become an acupuncturist. The other group, and I am ashamed to admit it, were people I found boring: a man who never remembered if the previous treatment had made any difference, whose symptoms never seemed to change in the slightest, but who insisted on coming regularly; a woman who permanently needed to be convinced at every session that treatment was working, even though, with her condition, improvement was only going to be gradual at best.

What these two distinct groups had in common, of course, is that I wasn't paying proper attention to them. Because I was preoccupied with my own needs, desires and states of mind I couldn't see the patients properly nor could I hear what they really needed. Unsurprisingly, they didn't get better.

> Will not a tiny speck very close to our vision blot out the glory of the world, and leave only a margin by which we see the blot? I know of no speck so troublesome as self. (Eliot 2003, p.419)

I now know that my attention on my own needs can blot out the patient – a cautionary phrase for sure. And a philosopher of medicine comments: '...real compassion and real intuitive knowledge are functions of conscious attention, without which scientific information and altruistic emotions are blind' (Needleman 1992, p.85).

All of which is to say that a necessary condition for intuition to flourish is that you give your patients your closest, most acute and most dispassionate attention.

Perceptual skills

In any treatment, attention comes before anything else. As your patient walks into the treatment room your attention needs to be at work, long before you start to think about any diagnosis, let alone points. Then, as you look, listen and touch, you may be suddenly struck by the fact that your patient is not telling you something crucial – and you may even be able to surmise what it is – or you may see a flicker of fear in his eye when he thinks you aren't looking at him or a cast of sadness may lie for a moment on his face.

'Sometimes it's the first glance at a face when you might get a "hit" of a perception of a colour...the colour you pick up at that brief moment might not be physical but energetic' (Ballentine 1999, p.167). Or it may be that when you take the pulses or palpate a channel you become aware that it is the Small Intestine, for example, that is in need of support. In all these instances what is happening is not thinking but perceiving in the second way, the way that showed the full colour of the cyclamen. Then the perceptions lead to a diagnosis and then, following on logically, to a treatment principle and then, equally logically, to a set of points.

But sometimes the perception will be so compelling that these subsequent stages of thinking become unnecessary. The master practitioners I mentioned earlier had a quality of attention that was so clear and so strong that they knew intuitively what their patients needed and what points to do without going through the mental processes of diagnosis and planning. That is how they were able to work so quickly and so powerfully. This way of working certainly has its pitfalls, and I will come to them later, but for now I want to look at its potential. Here is a sort of thank-you letter, written long after the event, to the family doctor who came out to visit a small child, ill in bed at home:

> Your face is full of attention, full of listening. How I remember that face! No one ever looked at me or my body with such a face. How you trusted your power of listening, your state of attention. And how your trust brought into our house and into myself a movement towards a new order. (Needleman 1992, pp.3–4)

This passage speaks of the raw power of attention. Irrespective of the information it provides to the practitioner, it has a powerful effect on the patient. I am sure that the phrase 'a movement towards a new order' rings a bell with you. There will have been sessions in your treatment room when you felt that a corner had been turned and you sensed for the first time an unmistakable shift for the better. Some old stuckness had been loosened and, like a stream pushing away the debris that has dammed it for so long, a new momentum got under way. It can come, as in this example, not from any treatment but from the sheer force of the practitioner's attention.

It was this memory of his childhood experience that solved a puzzle that had been worrying the writer for years.

> Freud's theories of the unconscious were riddled with prejudices and naive metaphysical assumptions based on the then current mythologies of biology... How could a man whose theoretical constructs about the human psyche were so complicated and artificial be such a good physician? ... Freud was able to look at himself and his patients with a power of attention that is only rarely experienced in the ordinary life of people... The unbounded energy of attention

that Freud emanated to his patients was the healing factor. (Needleman 1992, pp.49, 54)

The focus of our training is normally on the energetic effect of needles and moxa, but the 'energy of attention' should be counted too. This is not some absurd new-age notion; modern science has shown that simply observing a system changes it. And it is known in the classical texts of Chinese medicine where it is called 'medicine without form' – without form because it needs no remedies or techniques.

> The immediate responses of the physician in the clinical encounter – the words, posture, gestures, questions, attention, intention, genuineness, empathy, compassion, belief, and vision – deeply affect and resonate with the Spirit of another human being... Qi Bo, the medical teacher in the Nei Jing, admits that his sage teacher not only was not dependent on normal diagnostic methods, but also had no use for routine therapeutic interventions such as herbs or acupuncture. (Kaptchuk 2000, p.290)

This is inspirational, but notice that there is a danger too; if attention can change a system for the better then it must be able to change it for the worse. It is not something we want to do, of course, but we might end up doing it by mistake.

How best to guard against it? Thinking about those patients of mine who did not get better, it seems to me plausible that because my attention had a crucial slant or bias, because it was used to try and get my patients to be, or do, or provide something, then that tainted it. Which certainly meant that I didn't collect the information I needed, and I think it was also why the treatments didn't work.

One implication of all this is that we can amplify the effect of our treatments by improving the quality of our attention. Apart from the obvious ways, like trying not to think of the letter you need to write or the fact that you forgot to buy tea on the way to work, there are two main ways to do it.

The first is to refine your perceptual skills. One of my teachers had a lovely exercise that demonstrated how to do this. He asked us to watch him walking across a room three times and write down what we noticed each time. The first time, naturally and without thinking about it, we all followed him with our eyes. Then he told us that the second time we were to keep our eyes fixed on one part of the room and see him only when he crossed it. The third time we were to look away, keeping the area in which he walked only just within the edge of our peripheral vision. The difference between what I noticed each time was astonishing. In the first it was pretty conventional stuff: the speed of his walk, the slight swagger of his gait, and there were thoughts about him too and memories of watching him at work – in other words my attention wavered and went elsewhere. The second time I got an impression of his energy: as he passed I could tell, somehow, that he was a little tired, that his normal ebullience wasn't quite as bouncy as usual. And the third time I saw a colour on his face that I had never seen before (and which I can now not see); a completely new and fresh perception.

We usually look at our patients with only the first kind of attention, and that limits what we can perceive. I use the third kind of attention often, and quite deliberately. There are plenty of opportunities in a session, but there are two times that work well for me. One is right at the start of when the patient is settling down in the chair and I pick up my pen and write the date at the top of my notes, taking care to keep his face in my peripheral vision. The other is after I have taken the patient's pulses. As I turn away to note down what I have found I let my eyes drift across the whole of the patient's body. Sometimes I become aware of something specific – a recent example is of a strange kind of contraction in the patient's left hip and shoulder. He hadn't mentioned a problem with either but it led me to ask if he had ever had a bad fall on his left side. But more often what I get is a general impression of the patient's energy. It doesn't come to me as a diagnosis, more as a quality. I tend not to put it into words, though thinking of some recent patients I could say that their energy was 'delicate', 'armoured', 'constricted' or 'off to one side'. At any rate I know that it is important information and that it influences both how I am with them and the treatments I choose.

As well as peripheral vision, there might be a counterpart with the other senses. Going back into the treatment room today after the patient had left, I caught a faint odour of which I had been completely unaware while we were together. It made me think of stagnant water. There was no obvious connection with what I had seen in him so far, but next time I'll look more closely and pay more attention to the energy of the Kidney and Bladder. Then there is what might be called peripheral sound. I remember a patient's voice that started a phrase with some force but by the end had tailed off into a mumble that was hard to hear. I thought this pointed to a kind of depletion in him, as if he had enough energy to start to communicate a thought but it ran out before he got to the end. Then there is a tone to the voice that may take you by surprise; a young man with a powerful presence might sound weak, irrespective of the content of what he is saying. Those who learn five element constitutional acupuncture are taught to pay close attention to these signs and to classify them in accordance with the phases or elements, but even without this training the fleeting impressions you receive can reveal something that a focused attention might miss.

The second way of improving the quality of your attention is to notice how you feel in the presence of your patient, for such feelings might arise from something that you have become aware of without realising it. This is an ability that is remarkably well developed in medical intuitives – people who have little or no medical knowledge and who have been given no information about the patients' signs and symptoms, and yet manage to come up with an accurate diagnoses of their ailments. Just to show what is possible, here is a report of a study by an eminent neurosurgeon. The woman he writes about never met any of the people whose conditions she diagnosed, and was only told their names and dates of birth.

> Just how good is Caroline as an intuitive diagnostician? In this section, we will present data which indicates she is 93% accurate... I can only conclude...that any physician who, at the conclusion of an initial history and a physical exam, is as accurate as Caroline with just a name and a birthdate, would be one of the most revered diagnosticians of all time! (Shealey and Myss 1988, pp.74, 83)

As far as I can tell, these medical intuitives all work in different ways, but some of what they report can be used, in principle and in a suitably watered-down form, by any practitioner. Commonly, they speak of being acutely aware of their own responses to the patient. Psychotherapists are well aware of the phenomenon and call it counter transference. I am too sure that all acupuncturists have felt a sudden and unaccountable emotion in the presence of a patient; I have one who makes me angry for no apparent reason and I am pretty sure that it is because his Liver and Gall Bladder are constantly calling out for attention and asking (or rather demanding) that I get the message. It isn't hard to see how this works.

> ...think of the difference between the feelings you would sense from a person who loves you and the feelings you would sense from someone who is angry with you. No words would need to be exchanged since the quality of the vibrations being transmitted by both individuals would

easily be understood at the intuitive level... Intuition is
your emotional apparatus upgraded to a perceptual skill.
(Shealey and Myss 1988, pp.92, 85)

In other words, the kind of everyday empathy we can each
feel with another human being can open us up to a deeper
understanding of his condition. I sometimes find myself with
odd pains or sensations in my body during a treatment, and I
think I might be sensing 'the quality of the vibrations' of my
patient's pain or discomfort. A much more precise and powerful
example comes from Fritz Smith. Once, when holding his
patient's hip joint under slight tension, he said, 'From here I
can navigate around the body', by which he meant that he could
get a sense of the state of the patient's energy in the different
organs. I remember thinking at the time, 'Oh really? You might
be able to but I'm sure I can't.' And then one day, many years
later and largely, I am sure, because he had opened me up to the
possibility, I had a similar awareness with a patient. It was a kind
of empathetic understanding, almost a recognition – 'Oh. So
that's what it is like to be in that body!'

The wife of a Chinese acupuncturist gets worried when her
husband does this kind of thing.

> Qiu's wife was concerned...she knew that her husband could
> develop such empathy for his patients that he would take on
> their ailments during the process of healing, particularly if
> the problem was very difficult to solve. (Hsu 1999, p.35)

If Qiu can do that then he is getting very direct intuitive
information about his patients' problems – their nature,
location and severity. This is beyond most of us, but we do
sometimes have a response to our patients that is quite different
from deciding, for example, that a patient is deficient in Spleen
Qi, and I think it can give us a profound form of knowledge.

Today I treated a woman who suffers from quite marked bloating under the rib cage and gets sore breasts for about ten days before her period. I don't know what it feels like to be her and I don't need to know because the theory and concepts of Chinese medicine provide a perfectly adequate diagnosis. But with another patient who suffers from quite violent acid reflux, I get a very clear sense of a kind of self-abnegation, which turns her inwards, makes her tight and anxious and leaves her unable to take in what she needs. This insight came not from theories or concepts but from my felt experience. Because there is some fellow feeling between us, even if it is only partial and superficial, I can identify with her plight. In fact, I am not at all sure that I would have been able to treat her properly without it, nor can I see how a diagnosis along normal lines would capture her unique energetic state. Maybe I am exaggerating, but I think it would take quite a lot of distortion to fit her into any of the standard categories. I am sure you can think of patients like this, people to whom you respond by finding unusual diagnoses and doing treatments that may surprise you even as you do them.

Spirit

In an age when Western medicine offers so many successful treatments for physical ailments, many of our patients come to us because they have some awareness that the disturbances and distortions under which they are labouring are fundamentally troubles of the spirit. They don't have to be spiritual people to know it; here is an example, not from a new-age therapist but from a soldier who escaped from a prisoner of war camp in Italy and had then lain hidden for many weeks in a cave.

That night something happened to me on the mountain. The weight of the rice coupled with the awful cough which I had to try and repress broke something in me. It was not physical; it was simply that part of my spirit went out of me, and the whole of my life since that night it has never been the same again. (Newby 1975, p.216)

Through shock or trauma, under great strain or from feeling acute shame, grief or disappointment, something inside can break. As we all know, acupuncture can treat it. And that is because, at root, the distinctions that are drawn between body and spirit are false. For William Blake, 'Man has no body distinct from his soul for that called body is a portion of soul discerned by the five senses...' (Blake 1975, p.xvi). And here is a very different man writing over a hundred and fifty years later: '...the spirit is the life of the body seen from within, and the body, the outward manifestation of the spirit – the two being really one...' (Jung 1985, p.253).

I know it is true but I still find it enormously challenging. It is so hard to live up to. Yesterday I had one patient with a lingering cough and another with a sore shoulder and I don't think I paid any attention at all to their spirits. Even now, thinking back, I only have a very vague and general impression of them, certainly not enough to be useful. And yet the spirit can be perceived when palpating a point or taking the pulses just as by looking deeply into the patient's eyes. Equally, a physical complaint whose aetiology or pathology has eluded rational understanding can suddenly be seen as the manifestation of a specific spiritual crisis.

So how can I not have noticed the spirits of these patients? What is difficult, I think, is to maintain a quality of attention that is genuinely open, that has a wide focus and that is willing to engage with what cannot easily be put into words.

...it will intrigue you to realise that empirical medicine, medicine based on the revolutionary act of looking attentively at what is right before one's eyes, springs from the greatest mystical teachings. It will intrigue you to realise that faithfulness to the visible world springs from faithfulness to the invisible world. (Needleman 1985, pp.10–11)

In other words, I would have done a better treatment for the cough and the shoulder had I remained faithful to the invisible world. This shouldn't be a surprise really because it is no more than the Yellow Emperor's physician taught all those centuries ago. 'In order to make acupuncture thorough and effective one must first cure the spirit' (Veith 2002, pp.215–16). Helpfully, he goes on to talk about the kind of attention that is needed:

The spirit cannot be heard with the ear. The eye must be brilliant of perception and the heart must be open and attentive, and then the spirit is suddenly revealed through one's own consciousness. It cannot be expressed through the mouth; only the heart can express all that can be looked upon. If one pays close attention one may suddenly know it. (Veith 2002, p.222)

This beautiful passage gives us both a lofty aspiration and a clear instruction. Because the spirit 'cannot be heard with the ear' we can't come to know it through words and concepts. Our eye must be 'brilliant of perception', which surely means that we must look without any agenda or assumptions and, most important of all, without wanting anything for ourselves – for there is 'no speck so troublesome as self'.

And then he refers to the heart. Sitting in front of us, our patients try to tell us who they are, what they amount to and what has brought them for treatment; and almost all of the time these messages are expressions of their personality. One will shrug off an operation that went badly wrong and has left her with permanent back pain and insists she is going to walk the Camino path for a whole six weeks. Another will complain that she feels terrible because she was on a plane yesterday that had to wait for half an hour on the tarmac after it landed, and she was sure something was desperately wrong and it's left her with a headache, and she is so busy at work – and so on and so on. Our patients' responses to life and its capricious ways do tell us something about them, but we can easily come to believe that this is who they really are; especially if we feel respect and admiration for the first patient and a certain impatience with the second. But our hearts, if we allow them to be 'open and attentive', may see them differently. They may notice a steely determination in the woman walker which, while it has enabled her to cope with a dreadful blow and a chronic impairment, has also hardened her and left her spirit caged. Equally, the heart may know that the nervous passenger is perfectly comfortable with herself, smiles at the fact that she likes to exaggerate her difficulties and can see that she goes through life with an untroubled spirit.

And finally there is sometimes a need to pay attention to your own spirit. I am sure that I work better when it is clear and untroubled, and on those days when I know it has been disturbed I realise I have to do some kind of meditative practice before I get into the treatment room. What I have discovered over the years is that it always seems to end up bringing my attention to the state of my Pericardium.

We all know that the Pericardium can be open or closed – energetically that is – or somewhere in between. For me, there are times when it is pretty closed, perhaps because I had recently been hurt emotionally but sometimes for no better reason than that I was in a hurry getting to work and there were lots of people dawdling on the pavement and getting in my way. So as I arrive at my treatment room I need a reminder to open it. The author Robert Heinlen coined a wonderful verb, to 'grok'. It means seeing, understanding, knowing, realising, appreciating, recognising, acknowledging – all at once. When my Pericardium is closed I can think about my patients, but when it is open I can grok them.

You may think it fanciful to talk of opening the Pericardium as if it were a garage door or a tin of tomatoes, but the old adage that 'energy follows thought' points the way. You can do it by thinking that is what you are doing. If you put your attention on your chest – it's the power of attention again – and perhaps take one or two slightly bigger breaths so that you have a body-felt sensation of the energetic shift as well, then you can feel a softening, a relaxation and a slight warmth that signals the change.

A word of caution is in order too. One day I saw a patient whom I had treated for many years and who had become a dear friend, so naturally my heart was wide open when he was with me. It was still open when he left and the next patient came in: a woman in a very disturbed state. A saint would have kept his Pericardium open, no doubt, and that might have been powerfully therapeutic, but the Chinese acupuncturist's wife quoted above was absolutely right to be aware of the dangers of doing so. A very troubled spirit can be contagious for us ordinary mortals and there are times when it is sensible to have the protection of a closed, or relatively closed, Pericardium.

And how do you close it? In the same way that you can open it – by paying attention. Instead of a relaxation and an opening, think of a tightening and a closing. It works. The energy of attention is real and it is powerful.

CHAPTER 3

Energy

With new patients you set out on a voyage of discovery. You seek to discover what they really need, knowing full well that sometimes they can't tell you what it is, and you make a start on trying to understand how their energy is failing to support them fully. They give you clues, of course, but they are often confusing, misleading or hard to decipher. And in any case you are trying to do something that is fundamentally difficult. You are trying to see the immanent and the unmanifest; the afflictions of energy, its excesses, deficiencies and imbalances, its vibrations and blockages, the distortions to its natural channels and flows – all pathologies that will have affected the minds and bodies of the people who have come to you for help.

Fortunately we can draw on the remarkable work of the great physicians and clinicians who have gone before us and handed down detailed descriptions of the functions and pathologies of energy. They have taught us, for example, that the Liver smooths the Qi, an insight of genius that enables us to identify and treat all manner of conditions. They also gave us the resonances of the five phases or elements, so that we can treat constitutional energetic imbalances. All of this is essential and invaluable knowledge for any practitioner, but however good it is, there is always a gap between these generalisations and the energetic state of the individual patient. Granted that you might see unmistakable signs of Liver Qi Stagnation, or an Earth constitutional type, still the fact remains that the patient is neither the syndrome nor the diagnosis.

This might sound like a rather pious exhortation to value the uniqueness of each patient, an ideal that is then forgotten in the search for a plausible treatment. On the contrary: it is at the core of the medicine we practise. Ted Kaptchuk is typically stern about this: 'For the Chinese, a pattern or diagnosis is mainly an emblematic category...it is not meant as a label for people' (Kaptchuk 2000, p.176).

How easy it is to forget. How easy it is to classify our patients as we read a list of syndromes causing dizziness and decide which one fits best, or ponder whether or not our patient's evident frustration comes from a Wood or an Earth imbalance. How easy it is to become so absorbed, as I do, in puzzling out these things that you forget the primary task, the necessary condition for any successful treatment, which is to meet each individual patient in her individual experience of illness.

> When one begins as a young doctor, one's head is still full of clinical pictures and diagnoses. In the course of the years, impressions of quite another kind accumulate. One is struck by the enormous diversity of human individuals, by the chaotic profusion of individual cases, the special circumstances of whose lives and whose special characters produce clinical pictures that, supposing one felt any desire to do so, can be squeezed into the straitjacket of a diagnosis only by force. (Jung 1971, p.548)

Coming from a man whose collected works about people and clinical practice runs to eighteen volumes, his last words are particularly alarming. Are we guilty of squeezing our patients into a diagnosis? Can we afford to ignore his fundamental point about diversity? After all, it is absolutely in line with the latest of scientific medicine: 'In the end, cancer genome sequencing validates a hundred years of clinical observation. Every patient's cancer is unique because every cancer genome in unique' (Vogelstein, cited in Mukherjee 2011, p.452). And more generally, 'anatomical individuality does not stop at faces and fingerprints: it extends to internal anatomy... People are biochemically unique too' (Weil 1983, p.57).

But what are we to do if any attempt to make a diagnosis distorts the reality of our patients? How can we even choose points? I wouldn't be surprised if you are feeling a little uncomfortable at the implications of Jung's view, but here is a cancer doctor taking it a step further:

> When I was originally trained in pediatrics, the method was simple and straightforward. You walked in, made a diagnosis, decided what was needed and provided it. The focus was on what you as the physician thought, perceived and decided... That's the standard medical disease model... Since then I've discovered that basically I don't know what's needed... I used to be ashamed of not being able to provide a cognitive framework or justification for my interventions. I don't feel that way any more. (Remen 1989, pp.94–6)

Can we really do without the categories we use every day, the methods by which we arrive at a treatment plan? A very well-known acupuncturist, founder of a college in New York and author of half a dozen books, seems to think so: 'Rather than search for a diagnosis, which separates patient from practitioner while establishing the unequal authority of the latter, I seek simply to connect with the patient at the point where he or she is stuck' (Seem 1997, p.359).

You might be happy to applaud the sentiments but find them unhelpful when faced with headaches and back pain, eczema and menstrual problems. I am certain that these authors are perfectly sincere and that they are all able to work in exactly the way they say, but none of them, as far as I know, has really set out how they do it. And I suspect it is because, with all their years of accumulated experience, they have ended up working intuitively with energy.

Movement

We usually diagnose energy by drawing inferences from the patient's signs and symptoms. But we can also perceive energy more directly by noticing movement or the lack of it. Synonyms for energy include animation, dynamism, liveliness, drive, force and power, all words that speak of movement; we see all of these in our patients as they manifest on physical, emotional and spiritual levels. I have a seventy-five-year-old patient who should be jetlagged the day after a twelve-hour flight back from her holiday, but who drives two hundred miles and then gives a lecture to a packed hall – and she drives back the next day to give another one. We also see the opposite; where energy that doesn't move becomes pathological. So noticing stuckness, rigidity, tension, tightness, compression or stagnation can lead us directly both to a diagnosis and to an appropriate treatment.

The way a person moves can be terribly revealing; there is a kind of nakedness about it. I am thinking of a tall young man who walked in looking like one of those toys whose limbs are joined by slack elastic; the splaying movement in his hips, shoulders, elbows, ankles and wrists was astonishing. And then there was the person who nodded at everything she said, but not at anything I said, even when (deliberately – just to see) I agreed with her enthusiastically. I remember too the woman who, as she spoke, put her hand to her face, index finger over the mouth like a moustache and the other fingers covering her lower lip and chin. She seemed to be hiding her words even as she uttered them.

...a lot can be learned about a pain from the way in which a patient points to it. Apart from saying something about where it is, the movement of the hand is often a tell-tale sign of its quality: if someone has angina, he often presses the front of his chest with a clenched fist; the whole fist shows that the pain is widespread; the fact that the fist is clenched tells us that the pain has a gripping quality. The pain from a peptic ulcer is often closely localised, and the patient usually tells you by delicately pointing to it with the tip of his index finger. (Miller 1978, p.146)

Notice, too, the energetic difference between a clenched fist and a pointed finger. The first is a movement of contraction and tension, of holding, strain and effort. A pointed finger on the other hand is an energy whose intensity is not contained but is directed outward in a targeted line.

Contraction and expansion represent the fundamental opposites of movement, and when they alternate they become the rhythm of life. The heart expands and contracts rhythmically, as do the lungs. We pick up these rhythms at the pulse, but I think we also notice them, perhaps less consciously and with less discrimination, just by being aware of the patient. We ask a question that appears innocuous but see that the patient immediately stops breathing as if he has been shocked. Similarly, we can't help but register if a patient is taking shallow breaths high in the chest, and we might sense that her energy is shaky, disturbed and somewhat fragile. By contrast, the energy of a patient whose breathing is slow and steady is likely to be stable and robust. This is reliable information, and with each of these patients we would immediately start to think of totally different treatment principles and different points, long before getting round to anything that might be called a diagnosis.

Also reliable is the information we gather as the rhythm changes. This can happen when we ask a question that touches some area of pain or distress, and even if the patient finds words that seem to dismiss or minimise it, nevertheless a sudden and involuntary alteration in the rhythm of the breath may tell a different story. And then there are the changes in breathing during a treatment. Often as the needle touches the point the patient will go very still and her breathing may stop or become very light indeed; then, after a much longer time than normal, comes a much bigger breath than normal. Fritz Smith has an explanation for this common phenomenon. He believes that when we breathe in we are taking in energy as well as air. As we are needled we get energy from the activation of the point, so, briefly, we don't need energy from the breath. Hence the pause. Then, sooner or later, the body has to take in oxygen and exhale carbon dioxide and it needs an especially big breath to do so.

So when I needle and see no change in the patient's breathing I suspect that I have missed the point; or, also a distinct possibility, I have chosen the wrong point and needling it has made no difference at all to the patient's energy. By contrast, there are those lovely moments when a soft, wide smile breaks out on the patient's face as soon as the needle touches the point. The smile is another kind of movement, of course, and one that tells of a benign energetic change.

I think it is helpful to see the two movements, expansion and contraction, as the eternal alternation of Yin and Yang. So when a patient tells me that she has just come home from a week away teaching children to write creatively, that they loved it and that the classes got bigger day by day as the word spread that it was tremendous fun (for the teachers as well as the pupils), then I am alerted to the impending change. After all this energetic expansion there must be a contraction; after all that Yang there must be Yin. Surely she will need to rest and she may feel very flat. So perhaps I can devise a treatment that will make the transition smoother than it would otherwise have been; perhaps I can warn her not to over-interpret the contraction, knowing that she might take it to mean that her normal life is inadequate or unsatisfying when it is simply an inevitable energetic rebalancing.

Rhythms such as these take place over a relatively short space of time, but people have habits of movement, or of rigidity, and over many years these harden into the posture of the body – which is a kind of frozen movement. It is a bit like the way a twisted tree trunk has been formed by some spiral in the energy that grew it. So by paying attention to the way a patient holds her body we can infer the energetic patterns which must have made her do it. Ida Rolf makes the general point, and puts it in context:

> Twentieth Century medicine, which has worked so many miracles, has been chemically, not structurally orientated... But any mirror or photograph would reveal that a great many problems are matters of...a three dimensional body fitting very badly into a greater material universe (the earth), which has its own energy field (gravity)... Looking at bodies that have been organised according to these premises you can almost see the lines of force defining the energy field that is a man. (Rolf 1977, pp.17–18)

Posture is almost like a signature or a fingerprint. I have some patients, I am sure you do too, whose posture is so eloquent that it tells virtually the whole story of the gradual energetic distortion that has created their current imbalance and that therefore suggests the kind of treatment that will be needed to rebalance it. In one patient, the discrepancy between a tense and contracted right side and a flabby and practically lifeless left side of the body was so pronounced that I was not at all surprised by the location and severity of her symptoms. And it was immediately obvious that whatever else was needed, the

first priority of treatment was to disperse energy on one side
and tonify it on the other.

Another patient, a man in his mid-forties, came into my
treatment room and stood to attention – his shoulders thrust
back, his head and chin forward, forcing an exaggerated curve
into his lumbar spine; then there was the young woman who
shuffled in like a nervous eighty-year-old; or the man who was
so still in his chair that the whole room seemed to freeze. In
all these cases it is tempting to see the patient's posture as the
expression of a psychological or emotional state, and indeed it is
unrealistic to draw tight boundaries between energy, structure
and psyche.

> Feldenkrais called attention to the fact that all negative
> emotional expressions are accompanied by a shortening of
> flexor muscles... The energy in a chronically flexed body has
> to work just to hold it up; the man continually has to add
> energy to the body to keep it going. Such chronic flexion
> gives a feeling of tiredness, of 'depression'. (Rolf 1978, p.39)

You may well have had patients with chronically flexed bodies
and you may well have recognised their emotional states, but
you may not have made the connection between the two.
As with all great teachers, Feldenkrais not only spotted it
but also managed to express it in such a clear and pithy way
that it is unforgettable. I doubt though that he worked it out
theoretically; more likely it came originally as an intuition,
which he was then able to explain and describe.

And this quotation points to the fact that much of the
pathology we encounter is to do with lack of movement; and
hence much of our treatment is directed at stimulating it:

> For the therapist of the psyche as well as the therapist dealing
> with the physical man, the goal is appropriate movement.
> The psychotherapist senses immobility in the dimension
> of time rather than of space. The individual, bogged down,

unmoving in time, unable to escape from his infantile
or adolescent assumptions or traumata, manifests this
physically as well as psychologically. His lack of movement,
his generalised or localised rigidity, are unequivocal in their
statement. (Rolf 1977, p.153)

This is so compelling. We believe our system of medicine to be
holistic – that it does not separate the person from the symptom,
the mind from the body – so if in our approach to a patient
we separate her energy from her psyche we risk losing the real
power and potential of the work. And it is easy to do exactly
that when we use energetic concepts for one and psychological
concepts for the other.

In fact there is a danger in using concepts at all, an idea
beautifully expressed by the famous teaching – if you can't see
the moon in the sky, a finger pointing at it is a great help, but
don't mistake the finger for the moon itself. That is, the words
and concepts with which we describe and talk about energy, or
psyche, are fingers pointing at the moon; they are not the reality.
Your own intuitive experience of your patient's energy may give
you a direct understanding of the reality – one unmediated by
the generalisations and ambiguities of language, by the different
schools of acupuncture or the separation between academic
disciplines. For one of the joys of working with intuition,
though it is not without its own dangers, is that it arrives as
an understanding or insight, not as the outcome of a chain of
reasoning. The experience comes first even if it is later expressed
in words, to yourself or to others. Qi Bo, as usual, says it best:

> What you receive as messages, your heart will understand.
> You can then visualise the patient's condition in your
> mind. You can intuitively know what the problem is. You
> do not have to depend on language... If you are developed,
> you can pierce beyond the physical and know the truth.
> (Ni 1995, p.105)

Mismatches

Sometimes the pulses and tongue, together with what the patient tells you about her complaint, all suggest a perfectly sensible and normal diagnosis, but at the same time you can't help feeling that it doesn't quite match the individual patient. The dilemma, then, is whether it is better to apply the theory even though you aren't convinced or to abandon theory, trust your intuition and set off into unknown territory. At these times, a direct experience of the patient's energy may resolve the dilemma.

I recently treated a man in his early forties – tall, good-looking, very well dressed, with a powerful voice. He told me that his main complaint was that he slept badly. He also said that he had a strange buzzing sensation in his left cheek, which he was sure was linked to a rib that never felt quite right, although his osteopath could find nothing wrong with it. When I asked about his job I discovered that he had worked at a senior level for two big companies and had left after serious and rancorous disagreements with both of them. The specialised organisations in his field all knew his employment history and none of them would take him on after that, so he was now self-employed and his work was much less interesting and very much worse paid than before. He felt unsatisfied by his work but could see no way of changing things.

As he spoke I kept thinking of Phlegm. It was partly because he had taken up positions with his employers that he had then been unwilling or unable to compromise, but more because of a kind of dense and sticky quality to his energy. He moved slowly, and as he did it made me think of pouring double cream or something even stickier like molasses, and his replies to my questions were in sentences that sounded perfectly coherent when taken individually, but by the time he had finished what he was saying I found I was absolutely none the wiser. My questions were not so much answered as smothered.

So I expected to find a slippery and floating pulse in the middle position on the right hand and a thick, sticky tongue coat. He had neither. Because I couldn't find any convincing evidence for a different diagnosis I decided to clear Phlegm anyway and then see what happened. It was remarkable. As the last of the four needles went in (St 40 and Pc 5 bilaterally) he fell silent for the first time. His colour came up, as did his pulses. Then, after ten minutes or so, his pulses softened and eased and he opened his eyes and said, 'Very relaxing, this.' I saw him for about a year, during which time I cleared Phlegm fairly regularly, and he managed to get out of the rut he had fallen into and find new work.

I have often wondered what happened that first time. Did he indeed have Phlegm, but for some reason it hadn't manifested on the pulses and tongue? Is that even possible? Or did the needles have some other benign effect that was nothing to do with Phlegm? In which case I was very lucky, because I'd certainly never have thought of using those points in any other context. Certainly, if I had been in a student clinic I couldn't have defended my decision-making, as it didn't rest on any overall diagnosis but on an intuition of the state of his energy.

It is tempting to think that the role of intuition is to arrive at some diagnosis or treatment that seems to come out of the blue, that is unusual and original and that turns out to be remarkably powerful. But that is an overly romantic view. It can sometimes simply suggest an idea, as in the example above, or give a momentary impression of a quality of energy. Perhaps, when you have reached a diagnosis that makes perfect sense and you bend over to needle a point, it might make you pause, uncomfortably aware that there is something you don't really understand about this patient and her energy.

When there is an inconsistency between a plausible traditional diagnosis and your experience of the patient another option is to let go of the diagnostic categories and let your intuition lead you to a unique treatment. This isn't perhaps quite as wild as it sounds. In the end, all treatments consist of a number of points treated in a number of ways. A normal diagnosis suggests a set of points; intuition can also suggest a set of points. Given all you know about acupuncture, you can judge if your intuitive set makes sense and has some coherence, and providing it does then you can proceed with almost as much confidence as normal. I say 'almost as much' because the standard diagnoses do represent the wisdom and experience of generations of scholars and practitioners, so they tend to be reliable – though it is worth adding that they are only reliable if you have applied them correctly, and I know that on countless occasions I haven't.

I saw a man in his early sixties who presented me with a litany of complaints ranging from odd pains in his left thigh, to repetitive strain in one wrist, to difficulty going to sleep, to a peculiar kind of throat clearing, which, he told me, got much worse if he brushed his teeth at night – a curious observation. I could see no overall pattern to these symptoms, nor could I convince myself of any particular diagnosis. On the other hand, I had the very strong impression that his energy was dispersed and scattered. He travelled a lot in his work and had two current intimate relationships in two different cities at the same time. In any case I could almost see bits of him flying off as he talked; his descriptions of his complaints had a kind of throwaway quality to them and were tossed off rather carelessly, as if he didn't quite identify with them – and he did wave his arms around quite a lot.

I thought he might feel much better if his energy could all be brought back into himself in one place at one time. It occurred to me to needle Du 20, and that led me to think of matching it with a Ren point, and then I realised that both are on the centre line of the body. That became, if not a diagnosis, at least a coherent principle. I needled Du 20, Ren 24, Ren 12 and St 41.

Again, intuition took me to a starting point and then all the rest followed on through a kind of logical implication. It is this combination of the two kinds of thinking that is so useful, and through which, according to Jonas Salk quoted in the last chapter, we can 'achieve the wisdom we seek'.

Your energy

We focus so much of our attention on our patient's energy that it is easy to forget the state of our own. And yet it affects what happens in the treatment room. Valerie Hunt, an eminent professor of neurophysiology, conducted experiments in which she monitored separately the energy of two people in a room together and found that only rarely was each individual energy state unaffected by the presence of the other. It is interesting to have it confirmed scientifically, but it is after all a common experience. There are those whose energy warms me, so to speak, and others whose energy drains me; and there are many other possibilities. And as a patient myself I find that my own practitioner's energy has a lifting quality to it, so I find myself becoming more voluble than usual and more engaged with the significance of the events of the past month as I speak about them.

No doubt my underlying energetic nature stays the same, but in the treatment room I find that it shifts, adapts or changes to some extent with each patient. I may be more outgoing with one but calmer with another, and so on. I suspect it is because I am responding intuitively to what each person needs at that treatment at that time. Some practitioners may do this deliberately but I imagine that for most of us it is an instinctive process. And I suspect that when we do so we are unconsciously using some common strategies.

One is to mirror the patient's energy. It is tempting to do this with new patients as we seek to show that we are able to understand them and empathise with their concerns. So when a person comes in with a clear description of her symptoms, an ordered set of goals for treatment and a specific request for appointments at the same time each week I might well respond in kind, giving instructions rather than advice for managing symptoms and being unusually business-like about payment, missed appointments and so on. I assume that such a patient will appreciate it. And perhaps it also helps me to understand her energy; instead of it being something that I observe outside myself I can feel, at least to some extent, what it must be like to be powered in that way. I remember a famous and successful entrepreneur who had succumbed to pneumonia and wanted treatment to help her recover. I was astonished at how much we got through in that first session – a good deal of her history, a summary of the energetic nature of lung diseases, a brief comparison of the different theoretical bases of Western and Eastern medicine, quite a few recommendations for places to eat where I was going on holiday later in the year, a bit about the difficulties of managing social media and, of course, a treatment. For that hour (and only that hour) I experienced her speedy and relentless energy and realised that (although it wasn't for me) it was tremendous fun for her.

With patients who are stuck I think we can find ourselves manifesting an energy that will help them to get unstuck – and this may be as important as what we do with our needles. Although I am not usually aware that I am doing it I can sometimes spot what I am up to. I find, for example, that I have an urge to control excessive Earth energy. When a patient requires of me that I am nurturing and sympathetic I can do it for quite a long time, but when nothing is enough and the demand incessant then I find myself making up rules and demanding their observance. With one such patient, as the list of difficulties attached to each possible course of action gets longer and longer, I insist that he omits all but two of the options, then I point out the costs of indecision and give him deadlines. It may be crude, and there are certainly those for whom it would be unhelpful, but given that what we are trying to do, in principle, is to bring more balance to the patient's energy, then using Wood energy to control excess in his Earth energy is one way of doing it.

If I were more subtle I might instinctively use the Sheng cycle rather than the Ke cycle. That is, I might slip into manifesting Metal energy by seeking the essence of his concerns, offering genuine respect for the way he has coped with his predicaments and expressing some regret that there is no ideal solution and hence that, sadly, what he really wants is not possible, and so on. And if I were more subtle still I might help his energy to move not so much by what I say but by a quality of my presence. In this example I might quieten my voice and my gestures, allow my chest to fold inwards a little and withdraw my energy away from its embrace of him and bring it back within myself. For if he is unable to move out of that sort of endless circle that is so typical of those with a preponderance of Earth energy, and so self-sustaining, then by finding himself affected by my energetic state he may start to inhabit Metal energy himself. It is a bit like making a tiny breach in a dam; I could be opening a channel along which his energy can flow again.

When the authors I quoted at the start of the chapter write things like 'I seek simply to connect with the patient at the point where he or she is stuck' (Seem 1997, p.359), I think that they must be doing something like this. And I believe that most experienced practitioners do so too, even if they are unaware of it. This will be just one of a hundred ways in which their intuition, borne of long experience, leads them to use their own energy in the service of their patients.

Finally, if your patients can be affected by your energy, so the reverse must be true too. And given that people come to us in pain and emotional distress, bringing their worst fears, their deepest sorrows and sometimes their rage, let alone their energetic imbalances, this is something we need to take seriously.

Some practitioners I know do take particular care and use some ritual or protocol of protection before they start work. Normally, it seems to me, there is quite a lot of protection provided by the fact that we meet our patients in the role of practitioner, that we are in our own space, that we are in charge of the session and that we are at work – with our specialist knowledge and techniques separating us from our patients. Still, there are times when I rely on my intuition to tell me to take extra care or to take steps after the session to make sure that I shake off any energy that is not mine.

I expect we all have our own sensors, but I will describe mine in case it helps you to identify yours. The first is a very particular body sensation. I get a sinking feeling in my lower abdomen, near the anterior superior iliac crest on the left. It is unpleasant, as if there is something wrong there, some pathology. I can get it at any time in a session but it usually happens when I am taking the pulses on the right hand. I spent ages wondering why it felt like this and why it was in that place and realised one day that it was because one of my first patients was a very disturbed young man, probably badly affected by the drugs he had taken; when I took his pulses I mistakenly held his hand very close to my body just there and his energy invaded my own. Thanks to treatment from my own practitioner I got rid of it, but the memory is still there in my body. Nowadays it is benign; like the warning light on a car dashboard, it alerts me to danger.

My other sensor is also a body-felt sensation – perhaps the transmission of Xie Qi can't be registered by the brain. Anyway, it happens when a patient is talking about her life and I start to feel distinctly uncomfortable. This is quite different from an emotion I might feel when I am told something terribly sad or painful; that can be hard to bear but it doesn't make me wriggle in my chair or feel heat rising, nor make me want to look for an excuse to leave the room for a moment or even tell the patient to stop – all signs of discomfort. I think it happens when the patient is in the grip of an energy that isn't hers but is alien or foreign in some way; in earlier times it might have been called demon possession. And I start to be affected by it when I realise that the patient's view of her situation, and especially of the others in her life, is unrelentingly black. It is all doom and gloom; other people are all malign and the light has gone out. There is nothing good in the world.

Of course, such patients need our treatments and deserve our compassion, but as we minister to them we need to be alert, I think, to the promptings of our intuition, for it may be telling us to take care to preserve the integrity of our own energy.

In a way, this is to restate a theme that has run through the whole chapter. We can learn enormous amounts about energy in the human body from books and from lectures – where it flows and how it typically gets disturbed or distorted – but in the treatment room, in the moment, we have to rely on our senses to give us an accurate account of the energy of each patient. And what is sometimes called the sixth sense has a crucial part to play. It can tell us when our intellectual analysis is inadequate or wrong; it can suggest a way forward when we cannot think what to do; it can protect us from harm; and it can suddenly show us a truth we could not arrive at through any form of reasoning. And it can do all these things precisely because it is able to apprehend energy directly.

CHAPTER 4

Touch

Through the course of a single treatment we spend a lot of time quite literally in touch with our patients. We take their pulses, usually a number of times, and feel their bodies to find the points we are going to needle. If we are looking for a Back Shu point our fingers will first be on bone as they walk down the spine, whereas they press into quite sensitive soft tissue if we're locating Ren 4 or St 9. And some practitioners also use palpation of the channels or the abdomen as a primary means of diagnosis. All this distinguishes us sharply from most doctors. I injured my back very badly a few years ago and was taken to hospital in acute pain. Over the course of the next few months I saw six doctors of one kind or another, and not one of them touched my back; not one of them thought it would be a useful way of gaining information about my injury.

I couldn't help thinking what a lot they were missing. And what a lot we acupuncturists would miss if we do not make the fullest possible use of the times when we are in touch with our patients. For the messages that come from our patients' bodies, unlike so much of what they say, are not mediated by their personalities. Temperature or tension, dampness or dryness, skin quality and muscle tone all speak very directly to us. So too does the patient's reflex response to touch. I always remember the first time I palpated the back of a patient I knew well in order to find Bl 14, for he instinctively pulled away from my touch. There is a kind of truthfulness about the information we receive from our hands.

The touch of a person who loves and cares for us is so very different from that of someone who is angry, and I cannot imagine that we could mistake one for the other. Nor do we have to ponder whether the person we are touching is tense; if he is, we know it immediately. By contrast, our vision can often mislead us. We all know those pictures of lines that look like arrows, where the one that seems shorter is actually longer, and we all have had the experience of misjudging distances. I regularly confuse smells too. But when an experienced violinist puts her fingertip on a string she will know immediately if it is the tiniest bit misplaced. 'Suzuki knew from his experiments that truthfulness lies at the fingertips; touch is the arbiter of tone' (Sennett 2009, p.157).

And when I think about a patient's signs and symptoms, I can usually talk myself into one of a dozen diagnoses, all equally plausible. I can persuade myself that his response to my questions is aggressive when in fact he is simply shy, or that the colour I see on his face is yellow when in fact it is green. But I don't doubt the sensation of a velvety skin under my fingers, or a pulse that is full to bursting, because they are direct experiences. And then, undoubting, my intuition is awakened.

Here is a doctor of the old school reflecting on a lifetime of practice, and showing what can be done:

> I have never stopped trying to develop the sense of touch. Today, my hands are sensitive enough to tell you where you might have broken a bone many dozens of years past. I just move my hand down the limb until I feel a little rough edge, a drag in the muscles, and the added calcium that formed on the bone when it healed. (Fulford 1996, p.17)

Quite apart from the value in principle of having as many ways as possible of learning about our patients, even highly specific information, such as where a bone has been broken, can be very useful. Just recently, a woman I have seen ten or twelve times told me that she loved ice skating but couldn't do it any more. When I asked her why not she said that about four years before she had a bad fall on the ice, knocked herself unconscious and fractured one leg in three places, and since then she had lost her nerve for the sport. This traumatic event explained a lot about her and the state of her energy, and I would have been able to do better and more accurate treatments if I had known about it right from the start. She hadn't thought to mention it, but I am sure Dr Fulford would have realised as soon as he touched her.

Traditionally, the livelihood of all sorts of practitioners and craftsmen depended on the accuracy of the information they received from their fingertips. At a time when money was in gold and silver coins, it was vital to be able to tell the difference between the real thing and one that was made of base metal. The most reliable of all tests, in the hands of a skilled goldsmith, was the feel of the coin as he rolled and pressed and squeezed it; counterfeit money just didn't feel right. And the following quotation could almost be about what we do: 'The carpenter establishes the peculiar grain of a single piece of wood, looking for detail; turns the wood over and over, pondering how the pattern on the surface might reflect the structure hidden underneath' (Sennett 2009, p.277). Like the carpenter, we too are trying to perceive what is hidden beneath the surface, and we too can use our hands to feel where there might be flows, blockages or disturbance.

Which brings me to the whole business of what it is we learn through touch and how it is we learn it. For instance, when I take a patient's pulses I usually register what I am feeling in the categories I was taught – a pulse might be floating or slippery or full. But often these concepts don't quite apply to the sensation at my fingertips. So when I write my notes I find myself putting down things like 'Bold', or 'With a flicker on top' or 'Hesitancy on Lung'. Although this kind of information doesn't lead to a normal diagnosis, as the standard descriptions do, it is still extremely useful. For one thing, it serves as a baseline; so if, after needling, the pulse I have called 'Bold' becomes softer and less pushy then I reckon the treatment is heading in the right direction.

I also find that using my own language gives my intuition permission to join in and play a part in diagnosis. With the patient whose pulse had 'a flicker on top', I became aware that hidden behind his confident and urbane manner there lay a certain nervousness and a kind of fearful need to be seen to be stronger than he believed himself to be. And noticing a 'Hesitancy on Lung' led me to pay more attention to the quality of the skin under my fingertips and to become aware of a curious patchiness, for it was dry in some places and damp in others.

Another example comes from point location. There are points that can take me quite a long time to find, St 8 and Liv 8 are just a couple of examples, and I only know I am in the right place when I feel a difference in the skin under my fingers and some kind of yielding or opening in the underlying tissue. But sometimes, try as I might, I just can't find a point. I used to berate myself for my lack of skill, but nowadays I think it is because my intuition is telling me that there is nothing for me to do there; or, to put it more formally, it recognises better than my conscious mind that there is no energy available to work with at that point. So my mistake isn't in point location but in thinking it would be a good idea to needle that point in the first place. Intuition, arriving through or by the agency of my fingertips, prevents me from doing an unnecessary and inaccurate treatment.

> ...when qi stagnates or pathogenic qi invades from outside, the point becomes depressed or protrudes. Qi, which is invisible, is thus transformed into a 'quality' that can be palpated and distinguished. This is what is known as an active point, which serves both as a point for diagnosis as well as treatment... Active points manifest when there is some abnormality... In reality, there are no rules regarding how or when they appear. Some points appear right on the surface as if to say 'Come and needle me here!' Others are hiding next to a tendon or bone, while still other points seem to be holding their breath deep inside the body. (Denmei 2003, pp.5, 7)

There are many ways of recognising the feeling of an active point. Although I suspect that we all have to find our own way of doing it I have found it helpful to read a variety of accounts. The following quotation was written by a woman who was a research physicist before she became a healer, teacher and author:

> Another way to describe the feeling you may pick up from imbalanced points in terms of energy flow is that they will feel as if a little fountain of energy is squirting out of them or a little vortex of energy is going into the skin at that point. The same is true of imbalanced acupuncture points. (Brennan 1988, p.203)

Diagnosis

With a new patient, the initial handshake, the first touch on a pulse and the palpation of the first point can stimulate an awareness of the patient's fundamental energy state. This is so important. When I do treatments that don't help or don't settle well it is usually because I have misdiagnosed excess or deficiency, so I have tonified where I should have dispersed, or vice versa. Suppose a patient has good colour in his face, is ebullient, talks loudly and tells you how he really needs to do regular strenuous exercise – all signs of excess. How valuable it is, then, to see if his body, when touched, conveys the same energetic message. You might find robustness, strength and tension; but you might find instead flaccidity in his limbs, a lack of tone in the tissue and an overall quality of emptiness. That would prompt you to look more closely for other signs of an underlying deficiency.

Two famous practitioners write eloquently about this power of touch to diagnose. First, Moshe Feldenkrais, another physicist turned energy practitioner, and founder of the form of bodywork that bears his name:

> Through touch, two persons, the toucher and the touched, can become a new ensemble. Two bodies when connected ...by arms and hands are a new entity. Both the toucher and the touched feel what they sense through connecting hands... When touching...I only feel what the touched person needs, whether he knows it or not, and what I can do at that moment to make a person feel better. (Feldenkrais, cited in Johnson 1995, p.139)

This notion of feeling what the patient needs makes it very different from diagnosis by looking or talking, or by attempting to find a coherent pattern in the patient's signs and symptoms. In those methods the patient is an object, something studied. But through touch the practitioner merges in some way with the patient ('a new entity') and thereby has an experience of that person – at least in some way and to some extent. This may sound a bit far-fetched. But John Upledger, osteopath and

founder of Craniosacral therapy, believes it, and he adds a little
more detail:

> My own therapeutic style uses physical touch to facilitate
> the establishment of a connection between myself and
> the patient's unconscious. Other therapists may establish
> this connection by other means, but for me it is the act
> of touching, of physical contact between myself and the
> patient, that allows me to establish this connection. As I
> blend or merge with the patient by the use of touch, I make
> every effort to remain open to any perceptions, sensations,
> or insights that may penetrate into my conscious awareness
> from the patient... These messages may enter my conscious
> mind as pain in my own body, a visual image, a verbal
> message, or a sort of knowing or insight. (Upledger 1989,
> pp.70–1)

These messages he is talking about come to him in a variety of
ways, but none of them through reasoning or logic. They are
all stimulated directly by touch. And his 'sort of knowing or
insight' is an example of that momentary certainty that comes
unbidden and unannounced, which I earlier called 'sudden
knowing'.

In my experience these messages usually tell me something
about the patient's energy as a whole. One man has the massive
body of an England rugby player (which he was when a bit
younger) but his energy is delicate and needs to be touched
lightly, whether with hands or needles. And there was the
woman whose first few treatments consisted of points only on
the arm and upper back, all to tonify deficiency. So the first time
I palpated her legs to locate a point it was a shock to find that
her legs were heavy, full to bursting, leaden. I had assumed that
the emptiness I had felt before was her overall energetic state
and I had not realised that there was this mixture of fullness
and deficiency in her.

Sometimes the disparity is between the two sides of the body. Quite commonly I find that if I pick up each leg in turn, for example to locate Liv 8 or Ki 7, that one of them is far heavier than the other. On the scales, of course, they would no doubt weigh the same, but energetically there is a difference. Once when this happened I looked up and noticed that the patient's head on the pillow was way over to the right – if he were to lift his head and look straight down his gaze would have been somewhere outside his left little toe – so I started to think that the imbalance might run through the whole body. In an experimental mode, I palpated his shoulders, pressing them downwards first into the couch and then towards his feet, and sure enough his right shoulder was held tighter and higher than his left. All that made me think of treating the Luo points of the Yin organs on the left-hand side. I can't imagine that I could have devised that treatment unless I had received the initial message from my hands.

And rather like the peripheral vision of the last chapter, I think there is such a thing as peripheral touch. For example, when you take the pulses of a patient and feel that throb beneath your fingertips, your attention is sometimes diverted by a quality of the skin itself because it surprises you in some way. Imagine that you are taking the pulses of an elderly man, weary from looking after his invalid wife. They are deep and weak as you expected, but what really attracts your attention is his skin, which is damp, sticky and with a kind of film on top. It reminds you of a greasy pan that wasn't washed up properly. Given the weakness of his pulses, it might be hard to feel a slippery pulse, so you can take the condition of his skin as a clear sign of Damp or Phlegm. Or, to take another example, perhaps when you are trying to locate Sp 6 or Ki 7 you can't help noticing that whenever you press into the flesh your finger leaves a whitish indentation that takes time to fill again. So whatever other

diagnosis you might be contemplating, you know that the Yang
is relatively deficient.

And the same holds true after you have needled a point
or points, for you might notice a change in the quality of the
patient's skin. If it was dry, loose and a bit lifeless when you
first touched it and then becomes softer and warmer, you can
be pretty confident that you are on the right lines. When I am
unsure whether or not a patient has responded well to a point I
have just done, this can be a useful test.

> ...the associations between the skin and the brain are
> extremely intimate. This fact is the basis of the 'lie detector
> test'; specific mental states directly influence the electrical
> properties of the skin, and in regular ways that can readily
> be measured and correlated. And from blushing to hives,
> from goose bumps to shingles, the skin demonstrates a
> reflex expressiveness to scores of mental events. (Juhan
> 1987, p.35)

There is no formulaic correspondence between mental states
and skin condition, but if you can be aware of what you are
feeling as you touch then it keeps open an extra channel of
communication. At the most refined and profound level of
diagnosis those who use touch deliberately and consciously
develop a kind of intuition that bypasses the brain entirely.
Their hands appear to seek and learn autonomously or, to put it
more simply, they seem to have a mind of their own.

> In working with patient after patient...I find my hands
> almost moving by themselves. My hands move to certain
> areas of the patient's body...[which] may or may not have
> been related to my intended focus during that part of the
> treatment session... I learned very quickly to give my hands
> the freedom to go where they seemed to be drawn. I still
> watch in wonderment as my hands lead me to places in

the patient's body that I might not have found otherwise. (Upledger 1997, pp.6, 15)

This is from a man with a lifetime of experience and success behind him, yet he still watches in 'wonderment' at the workings of his own intuition. I enjoy the fact that it is still a mystery to him and that he can celebrate it in this way. He appreciates that it knows more than his conscious mind, and he has learned to trust it. Those of us who will never reach his level of skill can still take this as an exemplar.

Finally, intuition stimulated by touch can show us a way ahead when we can find no conventional diagnosis. Taking a patient's pulses one day I became aware that one hand was distinctly colder than the other. As far as I knew she had had no injury that might have affected the circulation or the flow of Qi in one arm but not the other; nor did I know of any theory that might account for this disparity. These are ideal conditions for intuition to flourish. In general, if we have a rational explanation for what we notice then we don't go looking for any alternatives, and in fact we may shut down the very possibility of alternatives. But when we are puzzled, or at a loss, when we have given up and admitted that we don't understand and don't know what to do, then there is room for some other voice to be heard, for some other faculty to exercise its own way of thinking and then it often comes up with an answer. When the constant chatter of rational thought stops, another part of the mind can do the work.

Therapeutic touch

It is not only the practitioner who gets truthful information through touch, so too does the patient. Our touch conveys a message, and the patient will pick it up intuitively and accurately.

In the early days of my practice, one patient, a good friend, was kind enough to give me the honest feedback that my touch was too cloying for her; she told me she felt as I was treating her as delicate and fragile, that it was as if I was trying to take care of her in a rather smothering sort of way and that she didn't like it. I was shocked. I had thought I was being sensitive and respectful, but apparently I was acting out some unconscious notion, no doubt learned long ago and never questioned, that this was what people wanted. After that, I came to realise that it would be far better to have a kind of professional touch; not harsh and impersonal, but with a kind of clear neutrality and unmistakable respect. And above all, a touch that felt good to the individual patient.

We have to use our intuition to tell us what kind of touch feels good to a patient. Certainly there are helpful clues: we might see a smile, or a grimace, as we pick up the arm and palpate to find Pc 6; we might feel a foot stiffen, or relax, as we locate Sp 3. One day, in order to needle Bl 60, I lifted a patient's foot off the couch with one hand and needled with the other, just a momentary tonification. When I took my hands away and told her that the needle was out, her foot stayed suspended in the air. I watched, fascinated, for a bit longer than I should, because I wanted to see how long she would keep it up. In the end I had to ask her to put her foot down. It wasn't hard, after that, to realise that she was quite extraordinarily tense and that I needed to touch her deliberately and firmly.

At the very least, if the practitioner's touch helps the patient to be relaxed and at ease then the energetic change brought about by the needles will have a far greater chance of flowing freely through the body, mind and spirit. If, on the other hand, the practitioner's touch leaves a patient stiff, anxious and expecting the worst, then it is easy to imagine an instinctive resistance to the needles and their work. But there is much more to it than that.

> As a physician, I was taught that you touched people only to diagnose them... And yet touch is the oldest way of healing... Marshall Klaus...was chief of the intensive care nursery where all the babies were these tiny little people you could hold in your hand. Each incubator was surrounded by shifts of people and millions of dollars worth of equipment. Everything was very high tech. Of course we didn't touch these infants because we'd get germs on them. But Klaus decided to do an experiment in which half the babies in the nursery would be treated as usual and the other half would be touched for fifteen minutes every few hours... And we discovered that the babies that were touched survived better. (Remen, cited in Moyers 1993, pp.355–6)

A scientist explains the underlying biochemistry (though it may only be part of the explanation):

> ...from my research with the endorphins, I know the power of touch to stimulate and regulate our natural chemicals, the ones that are tailored to act at precisely the right times in exactly the appropriate dosages to maximise our feelings of health and well being. (Pert 1997, p.272)

Given that touch in and of itself has this kind of power then we need to learn how best to use it and how best to tailor it to the needs of the individual patient. Only your intuition can guide you in this, although you may also need to test its reliability, which is the topic of Chapter 8. Your touch may be therapeutic, especially for those who are starved of touch in their lives, and it may also have a discernible effect on your patient's energy.

There are acupuncturists who are also bodyworkers, and when they take the pulses before and after a session of bodywork alone they usually find there has been a significant pulse change. Of course that comes after a complete or coherent treatment, but it isn't hard to see how point location on the upper back might help with constricted breathing or palpation of the Gall Bladder channel might ease feelings of pent-up frustration.

The following account sums up most of what is in this chapter. It was written by a surgeon, initially sceptical of acupuncturists and their methods of diagnosis, but who was astonished by what he saw when he witnessed one of the masters at work.

> Yeshi Dhonden...takes her hand, raising it in both of his own... His eyes are closed as he feels for her pulse... All the power of the man seems to have been drawn down into this one purpose. It is palpation of the pulse raised to the state of ritual. From the foot of the bed, where I stand, it is as though he and the patient have entered a special place of isolation, of apartness, about which a vacancy hovers, and across which no violation is possible. After a moment the woman rests back upon her pillow. From time to time she raises her head to look at the strange figure above her, then sinks back once more. I cannot see their hands joined in a correspondence that is exclusive, intimate, his fingertips receiving the voice of her sick body through the rhythm and throb she offers at her wrist. All at once I am envious – not of him...but of her. I want to be held like that, touched so, received. And I know that I, who have palpated a hundred thousand pulses, have not felt a single one.
>
> As he nears the door, the woman raises her head and calls out to him in a voice at once urgent and serene. 'Thank you, doctor,' she says, and touches with her other hand the place he had held on her wrist, as though to recapture something that had visited there. (Dass and Gorman 1986, pp.119–20)

CHAPTER 5

Relationship

I was often ill as a child. If you were unwell in those days the doctor would come to the house. I can still remember the rituals and ceremonies that accompanied his visits – the clean pyjamas, the tidied room and the appearance of the iconic stethoscope. Some of this was due to his medical knowledge and some to his role as the guardian of prescription drugs, but mostly it was because he knew how to help me through a succession of what we would now call psychosomatic illnesses, including asthma. His treatments were based on my need for respite and quiet as much as any medical diagnosis. We both understood that the decision to call him marked the boundary between health and illness and the beginning of a journey we would travel together until I was able to go back out into the world.

All this has been largely lost in modern medicine where cultivation of the relationship between doctor and patient might be considered useful in cases of chronic illness but as an unnecessary luxury in normal practice. You would expect a cancer surgeon, for example, to believe that accuracy of diagnosis and skill in the operating theatre are what really matter. But an eminent surgeon, though perhaps rather an unusual one, would not agree: 'I've become convinced that the relationship between patient and physician is more important in the long run than any medicine or procedure' (Siegel 1986, p.37).

Would I dare to say the same about what I do? Could I bring myself to prioritise my relationship with a patient above my pulse taking, choice of points and needle technique? Not without an internal struggle I couldn't. And it ought to be easier for me than for a surgeon. After all, the system of medicine that we practise recognises that what we are doing is to activate our patients' own innate ability to heal.

The quotation does force us to consider the reasons why the relationship is so vital, and it helps us to look for the ways in which it can be enhanced in order to amplify its power. The surgeon quoted above can't mean that any old relationship will do; he must be implying that it is one with particular qualities that helps the patient to heal (though he doesn't go on to say what they are). Another well-known doctor is more specific: 'I further believe that the art of medicine is the selection of treatments and their presentation to patients in ways that increase their effectiveness through activation of the placebo response' (Weil 2008, p.52).

The placebo response has a rather shady reputation. It seems to suggest that it doesn't matter what treatment you do as long as the patient believes in it, so why bother to learn all that theory and take the trouble to reach a coherent diagnosis? And, of course, medical research tries to eliminate it in order to prove that a drug has a genuine physiological effect. But if we see the placebo response as the patient's own innate healing system kicking in, then it makes sense to do whatever we can to facilitate it. The quotation continues: '...the best way to do this as a physician is to use treatments that you yourself genuinely believe in, because your belief in what you do catalyses the beliefs of your patients.'

I am sure that the vast majority of us take up acupuncture because we believe passionately in this form of medicine, so it might seem as if this key criterion is easily met. But there are times when it isn't so easy.

In my early days of practice I treated on the basis of the patient's constitutional type. I suppose I was right sometimes – after all, with only five to choose from, simple statistics would practically guarantee that. But even when I was right I was never sure I was right, and I now think that made all the difference. The same thing was true when I later qualified in traditional Chinese medicine (TCM). I would ask myself questions like 'Is this Liver Blood or Heart Blood deficiency?' and not know the answer. Or, when the patient showed plenty of signs of Damp, I wondered if it would be better to disperse Sp 9 or tonify Sp 6. Even when I happened to choose the option that my teachers would have chosen – the nearest thing to a right option I suppose – it was still the case that I was never sure of it. I was always conscious that there were so many ways to go wrong: wrong diagnosis for a start; right diagnosis but wrong choice of points; then right points but done in the wrong order or with the wrong needle technique, and so on. And every time I made a choice I couldn't help wondering if there was a better one I had missed. So I am sure that even when my treatments were good in theory, and looked sensible on paper, they didn't work well in practice. If I wasn't entirely confident in what I was doing, how could I expect my patient to be? And according to Dr Weil that means that I wasn't able to catalyse my patient's placebo response.

By contrast, we are given some wonderful moments, and many of them come, I think, from our connection with the patient's energy. Sometimes we are able to meet at a place that is beyond words and out of time. I once needled Lu 2 and I knew it was the right point because suddenly we were together, the patient and I, in a way we hadn't been before – an old woman who barely spoke, having long run out of the energy needed to form a sentence and who had so far accepted my treatments as an idiosyncratic gift from a devoted husband. For the first time she relaxed in my presence and her eyes sought mine. She seemed to recognise me. Unlike the nurses, the doctors and the physiotherapists, those well-meaning inhabitants of another world whose language she could barely remember and whose ministrations seemed utterly irrelevant, here was someone who had met her in her isolation.

Beginnings

It all starts right at the beginning, in that first session. Sometimes it may not be possible to form a therapeutic relationship at all. A young woman turned up saying she wanted treatment for a knee injury. I discovered that she had already been to a local physiotherapist, for whom I have the highest regard, and that he had helped her enormously with all sorts of pain and dysfunction, but that the knee was still troublesome. Why come to me, I asked, rather than continue with him? Why not stick with someone who had done so well for her in the past and with whom she had established a good relationship? Her answer was astonishing. She told me she was the 'advance party' for her husband. If she was able to give a good report of me and my work then he would want to come too. I knew then that I wouldn't accept her as a patient. As I treated her knee I would really be doing something else, perhaps even treating someone else, and I was sure that wouldn't work.

Sometimes it is less obvious. Rather perversely, you might think, in the first session I take almost as much notice of myself as of the prospective patient. Do I lean forward, engaged, or do I sit back in the chair while listening? And what do I do with my legs? Are they crossed, and do I swing away from the patient?

Am I bored? (I am usually fascinated, so if I find my attention wandering it's a sure sign that there is something unusual going on.) Am I untypically defensive about acupuncture and what it can offer? Am I suddenly clumsy? Do I feel unusually hot or cold? All these are indicators, for me, that my intuition is picking up something of which my conscious mind is unaware, and, what is more, something that might prevent me working well with that person.

I take especial notice too if I find myself saying something that surprises me. When intuition is at work the words just pop out. The first time I saw a young man in his last year at university he told me how difficult his life was because of his high levels of anxiety, which often affected his breathing so badly that he couldn't get out of a chair. As it happened I saw him at a time when I had no one after him, so I let him talk at length about the history of his complaint, which had been going on for four years, about what was happening in his life when it started and the way it had affected his hopes for the future. I heard about all the doctors he'd seen, all the specialists he'd consulted, all the tests and indeed all the complementary therapists he'd been to. His attitude to them all was somewhere between suspicious and hostile. In his opinion, none of them had succeeded and lots of them had been happy to send in large bills even though they hadn't helped him at all. When our conversation finally came to an end he stood up and asked, 'What do I owe you?' There was something about that form of words and the wider meaning of 'owing' that triggered my intuitive mind. It was because of that, I think, that the reply that came out of my mouth entirely bypassed any rational thought. I had no idea I was going to say, as I did, 'You owe me nothing.'

He later told me that this had made all the difference. In his mind, this set me apart from all the others and he was then willing to trust me as he hadn't trusted them. I am pretty sure that if he had asked instead 'What do you charge?' or 'Do you take cheques?' I wouldn't have found a way of saying what I did. What is more, there was a resonance about 'You owe me nothing' that carried far more meaning in his life than I could have imagined. (And, by the way, I did charge him for subsequent treatments.)

Similar, but more dramatic, are those occasions when you find yourself behaving somewhat out of character because you have picked up something that tells you to work differently. The last time this happened to me was with a woman nearing forty who was desperate to have a child. She had tried IVF and it hadn't worked. She was very warm and friendly, leaning in towards me as she spoke, smiling a lot and keeping eye contact throughout. She was enthusiastic about the prospect of treatment, which had worked very well for her best friend who had recommended me. She said that although she lived quite a long way from the clinic and she was busy running her own business, she was willing to come as often as necessary.

I was surprised to find myself being very tough with her. I asked if she could really cope with a child. Who would look after the business while she was having the baby, and afterwards too, when she might find it hard to concentrate on work? Would she go back, and if so, how did she feel about the child being looked after from an early age by some kind of minder? What was her husband's work and could they live on what he earned alone? I asked about the state of her marriage, and more. As the conversation continued, the bubbly effervescence died down and she started to think before speaking. After half an hour or so she felt able to comment that the session was not going as she had expected. She thought I'd be glad to have her business; it had not occurred to her that she might be a supplicant, let alone that I might not take her on at all. In the end, somewhat against my better judgement, I did take her on, but not for long. She cancelled her second appointment to go on holiday, was very late for both the next two – usually an indicator that treatment isn't going to work – and in the last of these she told me that she had gone to another clinic and was having drug therapy.

Perhaps I shouldn't have been so tough with her; perhaps I shouldn't have taken her on in the first place; perhaps, at some level, she was indeed ambivalent about having a child. But the point is that it is always helpful to look carefully at those times when your intuition prompts you to act in an unusual way. If it leads you astray then you might think twice the next time you are tempted to rely on it, but if it seems to have been accurate then it'll give you some insight into what you are really doing in the treatment room. Reviewing what had happened with this patient and looking at our interaction in terms of the five phases or elements, I saw that I had been trying to control her rampant Earth energy. It wasn't deliberate or even conscious, but I am pretty sure that I often work by responding instinctively to energetic excess or deficiency in the patient; had it not been for this particularly acute example I might never have found out. And now, when I start to do this with other patients, I can spot what I am up to and decide whether or not it is helpful.

Here is the same point expressed more generally and more profoundly: 'It seems that the closer our perception of self approaches the truth, the deeper our capacity for self-healing becomes… So the main responsibility of the therapist is to help the patient develop a truer, more correct self-image' (Upledger 1989, p.70).

If my intuition was indeed leading me to try and help my patient in this way, it was certainly not as skilfully done as Dr Upledger recommends, for he continues: 'The art of therapy is in sensing how rapidly the process can move without creating resistance or turning the patient away…'

Challenges

There are some patients, I expect you have a few as well, who challenge me in some way. Here are some examples taken from a long list: the patient who is regularly late for her session; the one who often forgets her cheque book or doesn't seem to have any money on her that day; the one who cancels about one session in three at the last minute; the one who always forgets to bring me the details of the medication she is taking; the one who starts practically every session by saying she doesn't think it is working (when in my opinion, and on any measure, her improvement is remarkable); the one who comments in a tone of voice overflowing with suspicion, 'My previous practitioner never did that point'; the one who has her hand on the door handle as she leaves at the end of her treatment and then turns back and gives me crucial information that, had I known it at the start, would have led me to do a different treatment; the one who always says she'll ring or email later to make the next appointment and then doesn't – at least not until she needs an urgent treatment as soon as possible. I could go on, and I am sure you could too.

Those who train to be analysts or psychotherapists learn how to work with these kind of challenges; for them the client is probably acting out what she will typically do in other relationships, so it is all grist to the mill. It is not so clear for us. Still, blaming the patient, getting frustrated or losing interest are not sensible responses, though I have done all of the above. One way of resolving these kinds of issues is to talk them through with colleagues, or even better with a supervisor, but another is to call on your intuition to help.

I am sure you can think of occasions when you've done just that. Faced with a challenge of this kind you responded immediately with something that changed the relationship in a flash; without analysing what was going on or what you needed to say or do in order to change things, you did exactly the right thing. The question, then, is how to get that to happen when you need it.

The key, I think, is to recognise when you feel stuck with a patient. When that happens it is because your normal way of thinking about what is going on isn't helping. The trick, then, is to cast the problem in a new way. Probably any new way will work and it doesn't much matter if it seems sensible or ridiculous; the point is that it might jolt your intuition into action. But there is one approach that is particularly appropriate for us acupuncturists and that is to frame the issue as one of stuck energy. After all, these patients come to you because they are stuck – whatever they have done before didn't help and they want a change in their condition – and if you don't find a way to cope with their challenge you will be stuck too.

You know a lot about stuck energy. You could ask yourself questions like: Is there a pathogen here that needs clearing? There might be Damp in the room so to speak, between the two of you, which is keeping you both passive and listless. Or you could ask yourself if you are experiencing some kind of Stagnation. The patient might be angry with you for some reason but be unable to express it overtly, so she is bottling up energy that is needed for change. And, of course, as soon as you ask questions like this then you will also be turning your attention on yourself and looking to see if there is anything in your energy or your behaviour that is keeping the patient stuck. Are you responsible for the impasse?

A patient I had seen two or three times turned up late without any good reason; in fact he told me without a blush that he had come out of his house on time for his appointment but there was a skip just down the road that had such interesting things in it he had to stop and sift through them, and one of them was so good he had to take it back home before coming.

Because I didn't challenge him immediately he never took me or my treatments seriously after that, with predictably poor results. Another patient was in great distress after a bereavement and I was naturally full of sympathy for her grief. That was appropriate for a while, but I kept on being sympathetic for much too long and it kept her stuck in her grief – at least while she was in the treatment room. I remember how astonished I was to see her one day on the other side of the street, bouncing along, laughing and chatting with friends. It made me realise that I needed to change my way of being with her so she didn't have to go on presenting me with the same old grief for session after session.

My final example speaks of the kind of behaviour we can get into when we treat fellow practitioners. One patient is a cranial osteopath for whom I have enormous respect; he has knowledge and skills I would love to have myself. I notice that with him I tend to talk less than with most patients for I assume he knows what he needs, can feel what is happening when I needle him and can make good decisions about how much treatment he wants. We get on well and he comes reasonably regularly, but I always feel I am not at my best with him and after he has gone I often think of the treatment I wish I had done instead of the one I did – always a warning sign in my opinion.

One day, as I moved his leg, I was aware that energy was being held in his left hip. 'Oh,' I said. 'I am sure it is completely unconscious but you seem to be holding onto your left hip.' In response he let go of the hip and a smile crossed his face. 'I expect it goes up to your right shoulder,' I went on – we both knew that holding it higher than the other shoulder was a habit he had long wanted to change. I went up to the shoulder and with very gentle pressure eased it back down. We paused and talked about the flows of energy through the foot, hip, sacroiliac joint and shoulder, about the meaning of holding a hip in the way he had and about learning to walk afresh. After that everything changed. Instead of deferring to his expertise and holding back on my own, which had created a gulf between us, we were together in the experience of a treatment and collaborating in the work.

All the difficulties I have been talking about are really difficulties of relationship, which leads to the question of how to avoid them. Or, to put it more positively, what do you have to do to enhance the chances of creating a genuinely therapeutic relationship?

Authenticity

If the patient is able to tell you what is really going on for her, to get beyond being charming or polite or interested or sceptical or gloomy – whatever it is she is accustomed to doing – then that will help you to work more accurately. So it is up to you to create the conditions in which that can happen.

Some aspects of this are the same for every patient. The treatment room, or area in a multi-bed clinic, needs to be a safe space, even a sacred space. Interruptions and disturbances convey a message to the patient that other things may be more important than her and her treatment, and who would reveal themselves in those circumstances? And anyone who has used a pressure cooker knows that a closed container amplifies the change you get from any input of energy. The old alchemists knew it too as they put their base materials into a retort. The treatment space needs to be inviolate in order to maximise what we do. It is the same with confidentiality.

On the other hand, each patient needs something different in order to trust you and reveal herself sufficiently for you to work well. It is a big issue, and I want to start to examine it through the example of prognosis.

Early on, many patients want to know what their prospects are, and how long it might take for them to get better: perfectly natural questions. Sometimes a general kind of answer seems adequate: explaining how the diagnosis gets more precise as a result of feedback from earlier treatments, how the work is cumulative as the body becomes more responsive, and so on. But sometimes that won't do. The patient needs more. Often, especially in the first few sessions, I don't really have enough information to be confident of a specific prognosis. On the other hand, I sense that only something quite precise and tailored to that individual patient has any chance of allowing her to trust acupuncture, and me, and hence to start the healing process. Perhaps you have encountered the same dilemma. Stay cautious and you may well forfeit much potential, or stick your neck out and risk the damaging crash of the false hopes that you have raised. And in the moment I am aware that the nature and quality of the relationship may well hang upon how this turns out.

I have had three kinds of experience. It is easiest when I just don't know. Then I simply have to find a way of saying so that isn't off-putting. Next is when I do have an instant and compelling opinion. It doesn't happen very often but I have come to regard it as an example of what I call sudden knowing, so I trust it and I tell the patient. It hasn't let me down. The last possibility is when I do have an opinion but it doesn't have that intense force of clarity and conviction behind it and I think to myself that it might be right, but it might not.

When this happens I ask my intuition to answer a different question instead, and that is: What does this person need from me in order to open up a little? Quite often I get an answer. Here are some recent examples: one young man needs to know that I appreciate what a hard time he had of it when he was a teenager and that I understand he is still suffering from the after effects; a woman with chronic migraines needs hope that change is possible and, as she is an academic, the best way to give her hope may be to provide her with a full explanation of the energetic causes; a teacher had to see that his panic attacks in the classroom came not from any underlying pathology but from utter exhaustion; and, finally, what was helpful with one patient was a new view of depression as an energetic imbalance rather than a psychological disturbance, because when energy is very low it is hard to find joy in anything.

Although there is a considerable variety in these intuitive responses, they are all essentially positive. Here is one doctor who came to learn the importance of this:

> I once treated a man in his fifties who had lived comfortably with a coin-sized lesion in his lung that was growing very slowly. After reexamining his old chest X rays, I told him that the lesion was consistent with a diagnosis of lung cancer. He was distraught to hear this. Despite having no overt symptoms in the past, he began to cough blood within a month and within three months he was dead. (Chopra 1989, p.183)

Another doctor draws more general conclusions from this kind of experience:

> Two years ago a man in his mid thirties came to me for a second opinion about his illness. After several months of worsening episodes of diarrhea and abdominal pain, his family doctor referred him to a gastroenterologist, who diagnosed the problem as ulcerative colitis and started the patient on a standard suppressive drug... The man disliked the side effects of the drug and did not think it controlled his symptoms very well...he persisted in questioning the gastroenterologist about other possible strategies, without

success. 'Do you know what the doctor said to me on my
last visit? He said, "Listen, I've got nothing else to offer
you, and, anyway, the chances are you'll eventually develop
colon cancer."' ... A high priest of technological medicine,
enthroned in his temple, had uttered the equivalent of
a shamanic curse, for doctors in our culture are invested
with the very same power others project onto shamans and
priests... I cannot help feeling embarrassed by my profession
when I hear the myriad ways in which doctors convey their
pessimism to their patients. (Weil 2008, pp.61, 64)

In addition to the damaging effect this may have on the patient,
such pessimism prevents the kind of relationship that is so
important for healing. The previous quotation continues by
referring to 'the problem of making doctors more conscious of
the power projected onto them by patients and the possibilities
for reflecting that power back in ways that influence health for
better rather than worse' (Weil 2008, p.64).

One obvious way of influencing health for the better is to
help the patient learn to manage her condition and to start
to change those behaviours that perpetuate it. A successful
course of treatment is a collaborative effort, so it is vital that
the patient plays her part. Some of my patients never manage
to do so, and it seems to me that it is because right from the
start I have failed to create the right kind of relationship with
them. I suspect it happens when I am not sure that I have
established any real connection between us and so I start to
shift and change what I say and do in order to make them
feel more comfortable. It's a trap; and I tend to fall into it by
getting carried away with the power of acupuncture, telling my
patient all about its fascinating view of health and illness, how
it can do things undreamt of by Western medicine, and how I
am the one to bring this good news to those who, at last and
after much suffering, have found their way to treatment, to the

gateway to a new world where all will be revealed and...and ...and more nonsense like that. As if I didn't know better. And so, of course, some of them take away the idea that acupuncture is so amazing and magical and they don't have to do anything themselves – even if I have said that they do.

Instead of concentrating on what I want to say I need to concentrate on the relationship, and specifically on how it can best be created with this particular patient. Normally, that shift of focus is all that is needed and from then on I can find better ways of helping the patient to help herself. In any event, this is not something that can be worked out logically; there aren't classical signs and symptoms, so to speak, of the different varieties of relationship from which I can deduce a syndrome, so I have to allow my intuition to guide me.

Endings

Finally, as with any relationship, yours with your patient is bound to come to an end sooner or later. It may all be perfectly straightforward because the patient has moved away or you both agree that what she came for has been achieved, but quite often it isn't. There are two circumstances that I have met a number of times where the ending has been difficult and where intuition can provide a helpful guide to how it can best be managed.

One is where the patient loses patience and opts for Western medicine instead, usually on the grounds that it will work more quickly. This can happen with muscular-skeletal problems where a cortisone injection promises instant and lasting relief (though it is pretty common that it only works for a few weeks); with chronic conditions like asthma and Crohn's (where suppressive drugs may seem to help, but can do long-term damage); and with depression. I want to discuss this last instance, though much of what I say applies to the other examples as well.

I have had the experience twice recently of patients who came because they were depressed, who had half a dozen treatments or so and who seemed to be getting on top of the things that had brought them down. Their pulses and tongues had improved markedly and so had their skin tone. Their withdrawn and somewhat crushed demeanour had disappeared and they sat straighter and looked me in the eye when they talked. In both cases I had thought that we had developed a good working relationship and had a mutual understanding of the process, so it was a bit of a shock when one rang to cancel her appointment, saying that she had been to the doctor and was now on anti-depressants, and the other turned up for her treatment but told me she couldn't go on as she was and that she had decided to go the conventional route.

The first task was to say something that acknowledged the ending of the relationship and left the patient with hope for the future. Not all that difficult, though given that I had clearly misread the relationship I chose to be pretty non-committal. After that I had to resist the temptation to blame some unknown friend or doctor for offering what appeared to be a quick and easy solution, especially when I didn't believe there was one. It was easy, too, to get lost in speculation about why each of them had suddenly called a halt. More productive was to pose the question: What did my relationships with these two patients have in common? And the answer came back almost instantly (as it tends to do when you hit on the right question): We didn't trust one another.

That was another shock for me, but I knew it was true. I realised that each of them would instinctively trust a doctor in a way they had never trusted me, and therefore, given all that I have said about the crucial importance of the relationship with the practitioner, I think they probably made the right decision. And if I am honest, I am not sure I trusted them either, for I suspected that neither of them would stay for long. Without mutual trust it is probably impossible to build the kind of relationship that enables healing.

It can also be difficult when the practitioner and patient disagree about the ending of the relationship. I am thinking here of the times when this happens in spite of the fact that a good relationship has been established and there is much mutual appreciation of the work that had been done. So how do you know when it is time to stop? And how does the patient know?

I had a patient who suffered from a very arrhythmic heart. Before she came to me she would be taken off to hospital in an ambulance every few weeks, and it was indeed extremely distressing for her, physically and emotionally. I treated her for a number of years, unravelling some of the causes of this condition, dealing with some other health problems and getting to the point where, when the arrhythmia happened, which wasn't often, it was only mild and she could manage it herself without treatment or medication. She had regular treatment every three or four weeks and, as with so many long-standing patients, it was a pleasure to see her. So why did I suddenly lose patience with her one day? There was nothing unusual about the session nor was I under any kind of stress in my personal life that might have explained it. But I had an overwhelmingly strong instinct that she needed to kick away this last crutch. I said I thought we had achieved what she came for and I wouldn't make another appointment; in case it seemed too brutal I added that if after six months she felt she needed a treatment she could come back then. Before the session started I had no idea I was going to do this, but I took my impatience as a clear signal that the work had indeed been done. She cried. I felt like a brute. But she didn't turn up again when the six months were up and her husband, who later came for treatment himself, told me that she is doing fine.

And then there are the times when it is the patient who decides to bring the relationship to an end even though you think there is more to be achieved. It can be very sad to see someone walk away when you believe you could really help, and I always wonder whether or not to put up a fight. One patient said he was leaving because acupuncture wasn't working; without pausing for thought I turned to the notes of our first session and read him the list of seven or eight symptoms with which he had arrived. He had forgotten them all except the one that was left. With another patient I suggested a small number of extra sessions with highly specific goals to be attained, as much as anything to give him a chance to reconsider. And sometimes my sense is there is nothing to be done except to say goodbye with warmth and good grace. And I keep a check on the accuracy of my intuition by writing on the bottom of their notes whether or not I think they will come back.

Finally, just as your skills in diagnosis and needling develop over the years of practice, so too do your skills in creating a therapeutic relationship. Some people are easy; I saw a new patient yesterday and in an hour we covered more ground than I believed possible, and we ended with much respect and affection between us. With most people it takes more time and patience, and with just a few it doesn't happen at all. In those cases, when no real relationship comes into being, I used to just carry on, concentrating on doing as good a job as possible; now I have become convinced that this is not really an option. And the experts agree: 'For some time I have been convinced that the common denominator, the golden thread that runs through all forms of healing, may be called the healing relationship' (Solfrin 1989, p.100). And: 'I don't know ahead of time what I am going to do in a session...but...the energy is always there – I trust that. It's always there but it's in the relationship, not in me' (Remen 1989, p.95).

You have to use your intuition to build a genuinely healing relationship. There are no syndromes and no manuals, and anyway it all happens too fast. The patient tells you about something that is making her anxious; your response can make her feel heard or misunderstood, seen or overlooked, accepted or criticised. Only your intuition, honed for sure by years of experience, can lead you to find just the right thing to say: something that is true, helpful and entirely personal all at once.

CHAPTER 6

Decisions

My practitioner allows the same amount of time for a treatment as I do, and yet my experience of time as a patient is remarkably different from my experience of time as a practitioner. As a patient, the session seems unhurried, quiet, even contemplative, and I often think she is giving me more than her usual hour, though she rarely does. By contrast, time flashes by when I am working and I am constantly surprised at how quickly the session comes to an end. I suppose it is because there are so many decisions to be made.

There is always the complexity of diagnosis and choice of a treatment strategy, and there are also decisions to be made all the time when you interact with a patient. One of them tells me she got cold waiting for a bus to come to the clinic; should I offer to make her a hot drink or will that change the dynamic between us? When, for the third time, a patient doesn't answer my question about when his pain started, do I let it go, ask again or point out what he is doing? A new patient's husband wants to sit in on his wife's treatment; do I agree to that or not?

And then there are the kind of puzzles you face when people don't respond to treatment in the way you expect. Take the patient I saw immediately before writing this, a man in his early sixties diagnosed with type two diabetes since the death of his much-loved wife, eight years ago. He was excited after his second treatment because both his insulin and blood sugar levels dropped markedly; there were changes for the better, too, in his digestion and his bowels. But the third and fourth treatments seemed to have had no effect at all and all the indicators returned to pre-treatment levels. At this, the fifth session, I could sense he was losing heart and that if nothing happened this time he might not come back again.

Here were some of the things going on in my head: Why was the second treatment so successful and why, by contrast, did the others have no effect when my treatment strategy was the same for all of them? Was there anything I could say to give him confidence in the process, and if so, what? It seemed as if the Kidney pulse was the strongest and had the best quality too, which was highly unusual – was I reading it right? Were the sessions having a cumulative effect, in which case should I stick to my original plan, or was it time to change tack? And (a very common thought) had I missed some of the points, especially Bl 20 (so the diagnosis might have been right all along)?

It is useful to consider how we make these kinds of decisions, and how we can improve our methods of making them. Simplifying drastically, the Western view of decision-making is very different from the Eastern. In the former, we are taken to be rational beings, which means that when faced with a decision we gather the relevant information, then devise alternative courses of action, then weigh them against each other and finally choose the best. It sounds fine, but I don't think it is what people actually do, even when making much simpler decisions than the ones we face in every treatment. For one thing, it is not obvious how you can tell when you have enough information, and in any case I don't think I'd ever have time to go through all that in a session.

The Eastern view of decision-making is very different. A witty example is the famous Zen story of the new and very keen young monk who enquired of his Master how long it would take to get enlightened. 'Oh, about fifteen years,' replied the Master. The young man was shocked; it seemed so long. So the next day he went back to his Master and asked how long it would take if he worked intensively, meditated for days on end and took no breaks. 'In that case,' replied the Master, 'it'll take twenty years.'

This is a version of wu wei, the Daoist notion of doing by not doing. There is a rich and enormous literature about this, and any summary does it an injustice. Still, briefly, the idea is that deliberately applying the mind and forcing it to concentrate with a narrow focus is not the way to get it to work well; on the contrary, that allows the ego to take over decision-making, which it will then do with over-confident bravado. Wu wei, on the other hand, leaves room for an unselfconscious and wholly appropriate response to what is happening in the moment.

> When a man has learned to let his mind alone so that it functions in the integrated spontaneous way that is natural to it he begins to show the special kind of 'virtue' or 'power' called te. This is not virtue in the current sense of moral rectitude but in the older sense of effectiveness, as when one speaks of the healing virtues of a plant. (Watts 1962, p.45)

This does have its appeal for acupuncturists. Under pressure of time, with so much to notice about the patient's words, behaviour, tongue and pulses, and with so many choices to be made about treatment strategies, selection of points, the order in which they are to be done and so on, this kind of decision-making looks eminently practical. And there is more to it than that. It is so easy, as a practitioner, to get lost in your own thinking, to be worrying about your diagnosis or trying to remember what your teacher said one day about what it means when the pulses in the first position are weak on both sides, so that you are no longer with your patient, no longer sensitive to his energy, no longer even in the room really. And if you are under stress like this with all your patients you will certainly get tired and depleted yourself, and that won't help either. Whatever its drawbacks, wu wei will keep you present and alert through the day and able to respond to your patients' needs. Here is an example:

> During this session which began like all the others, Qin suddenly interrupted the flow of his movements, took a needle out of the drawer of the table behind him and stuck it with an elegant movement and few words of warning into tingyang... I doubt that Qin knew from the start that he was going to use a needle. It was the only time I ever saw him resort to needling during a healing performance. The intuition that this was the right thing to do in this case remains a puzzle but it was by no means unique to this episode. (Hsu 1999, p.35)

The fact that wu wei removes trying and effort doesn't mean it is easy. It is, in fact, a form of intuition, and like any other seemingly effortless skill, it takes a good deal of practice to get good at it – though, of course, one of the delights of the concept is that if you work at wu wei then you aren't doing it at all. To be true to its spirit you have to practise by not practising!

Alternatives

A patient came to me two years after a complete and unexplained breakdown of his whole nervous system. Thanks to many weeks in hospital on more than one occasion, and a regime of powerful drugs, he was able to resume a pretty normal life. But he was left with some uncomfortable conditions, which his doctors said they could do nothing to alleviate. One was a chronic restlessness in his legs; another was an intermittent severe gagging when he drank – doesn't sound too bad, but when it happened he really didn't know if he'd be able to take a breath again; and the last was a loss of feeling during sex – he had no physical sensation at all. I might have been a bit unsure about how to proceed with these problems even taken singly, but I could think of no energetic explanation that might account for this peculiar combination of the three.

In theory, I could have fallen back on a root kind of treatment, but his tongue and pulses didn't suggest any obvious excess, deficiency or pathogen, nor could I identify a constitutional element or phase that was clearly out of balance. When the logic of diagnosis and treatment principles don't seem to apply, which happens quite often to me, then I have to make decisions in a different way.

I first take the opportunity to stop, to let my thinking mind quieten down, and then, sometimes, I can hear what the Quakers call 'the still small voice within'. Quite often I then become aware of a gap between what the patient is telling me and what I am feeling myself, and my working assumption is that it is because I am sensing the energetic reality behind the words. Some feature of the patient swims into focus and gains a relevance I had not appreciated before.

With a man who told me he was well and simply wanted treatment for a troublesome knee, I noticed a blotchy patchwork of colours on the face, which spoke of a mixture of excess and deficiency and which contradicted his insistence that nothing else was needed. Or, in one recent instance, as I listened to a perfectly sensible story about a patient's difficulties in looking after an elderly mother, I became more and more agitated and uncomfortable, and I realised that I was in the presence of a much bigger disharmony than I had appreciated.

Another alternative to the standard ways of making decisions is to ask for help. When my teacher retired he gave me a small bear carved of rose quartz – in his tradition this is the animal of healing made from the stone of healing – which he had kept in his treatment room for many years. It now sits in my own, and when I am at a loss I look over to the bear and I say, 'OK, I give up – what do I do now?' It all started one day when I was at a total loss, practically in despair (it can be quite fruitful to have given up completely), and the words just popped out of my mouth. I didn't expect to get an answer but one came, and I am no longer surprised when it does. A genuine cry for help, it seems, can shut down the normal thinking processes and open up the intuitive ones.

A variant of this cry for help is to go to a point that seems plausible at first sight. With the man with the three curious complaints I chose Liv 3 and palpated it. The idea is that my fingers will feel if it is what Shudo Denmei calls an active point. How can I tell? What does it feel like? I might be kidding myself of course, but I think that when it would be good for a patient I can sense a receptiveness, an opening, as if the patient's energy is readily available there. If I do end up needling such a point, it often suggests the next one. In this case Liv 3 could have led me on to all sorts of places like LI 4 or GB 34, but in fact it made me think of Pc 6, which I only then realised made sense because it was on the paired Jue Yin channel. And that led me to SJ 5, and so on. In fact, I can do the whole treatment like that, with no diagnosis, no theory, no treatment plan, just making one decision after another, swinging from point to point like a monkey through the trees (though unlike the monkey I do take the patient's pulses at each stage to check to see if what I am doing is working well or not).

It may sound odd, even foolish, to make decisions that don't arise from an application of the theories of Chinese medicine but it does have some merit when the normal protocols aren't helping. It stops me using a diagnosis in which I don't have confidence.

> I believe that the art of medicine is the selection of treatments and their presentation to patients in ways that increase their effectiveness... The best way to do this as a physician is to use treatments that you yourself genuinely believe in, because your belief in what you do catalyses the beliefs of your patients. (Weil 2008, p.52)

Another merit is that it makes sure that I pay the closest possible attention to the patient at each stage of the treatment. Before I needle I am on the lookout for the slightest sign of what is going on energetically, and after needling I am alert to the possibility that what I am doing isn't making things better – the pulses don't improve, the patient's colour stays blotchy or his voice loses strength and timbre. I was once asked to teach in a clinic where, after the students and supervisor had arrived at a diagnosis and the needling was done, the patient was ignored until it was time to take the needles out again. I thought it showed an unwarranted confidence in their decision-making because they simply assumed that what they were doing must be right. There must have been times when their diagnoses were wrong, or at least inadequate, but they would never have known, and they never took the opportunity to change a poor treatment into a good one.

With all these strategies, what I am really doing is creating the conditions for what I call unconscious inferences. My conscious mind hasn't been able to come up with anything convincing, so I am giving my unconscious mind as much detailed information as possible, and that in turn gives it the maximum opportunity to compare what I have in front of me with the lessons and examples stored in my memory bank. With luck, sooner or later, it will find a fit; there will be something that I have seen before and understood, and I will realise that it is relevant now with this patient. And sometimes, just pausing like this, just realising that the rational, deductive process that serves us all so well most of the time isn't helping, sometimes that is enough to open the door to one of those moments of sudden knowing, where doubt changes to certainty in a flash.

Collaboration

Talking about using intuitive decision-making as if it were simply a fall back and a substitute for the main methods when those aren't working does raise an interesting question: Does treatment based on tried-and-trusted methods of diagnosis – Japanese Meridian Therapy, TCM, Stems and Branches or any other – have a different power or quality from one based on intuition? In other words, is there more to it than just having a different way of deciding which points to needle?

In the standard medical model the patient doesn't know what is wrong with him, and even if he did he wouldn't have the expertise to choose or apply a remedy. He is passive, while the doctor actively sets to work to find out what has caused the patient's condition and what might be an appropriate remedy. According to this view of the process all the decisions are being made by the practitioner while the patient makes none. Our own experience tells us that this is unrealistic, and there are deeper reasons why it isn't true.

> The science of vibrations applies to all clinical methods. Regardless of the philosophy of the technique being used, intricate energetic interactions occur between nearby individuals, even if they are not in physical contact. Seeing

and talking with another person are energetic interactions, involving light and sound vibrations. (Oschman 2000, p.121)

Previously I pointed out that the state of your own energy will have an effect on your patient, and the question arises whether that effect will be significantly different if you are making decisions not by following the logic of a standard method but by intuition. If so, then irrespective of the points and needle techniques you choose, the two kinds of treatments may be very different.

I think there are a number of reasons to believe that this is the case. The first is that the patient's intuition is likely to respond to the activation of your own. The author of the quotation above would see it as a matter of vibrations, the way pendulum clocks on a wall end up synchronised, or women who live together find that their periods arrive at the same time. Whatever the scientific explanation, I have seen the phenomenon too often to doubt it. Recently I allowed my intuition to lead me in my first session with a woman who, because of her severe eczema and many allergies, was on a very restricted diet. I found myself saying that I thought she might do better with herbal medicine rather than acupuncture, and I also suggested it might be a good idea if she could give herself permission to go to bed for an hour when she got home weary from work. At one point in the treatment she suddenly said, 'I don't want to be on my diet any more,' and was astonished by the words that came out of her mouth. It had never occurred to her before, and until she said it she wouldn't have believed it possible. I cautioned her to be careful, but she looked at me with unmistakable shen in her eyes for the first time in the session and told me that she knew it would be alright. And, actually, I didn't doubt her.

> ...intuition is not mere perception or vision but an active creative process that puts into the object just as much as

it takes out. Since it does this unconsciously, it also has an unconscious effect on the object. (Jung 1971, p.366)

There is a more general lesson to learn, I think, from this. In an earlier chapter I spoke of the importance of collaboration, how the patient has to start to make changes in his life to support and amplify the treatment. But now I want to say that when the patient starts to respond, consciously or not, to your intuitive leadings, then something more profound starts to happen. A very experienced practitioner said to me that when she works in this way her needling feels like an invitation to the patient, one that may be accepted or rejected. If the former, she feels an instant response of connection; if the latter, she takes the needles out fast (though nowadays she is so well attuned that she usually stops herself the moment before insertion). When this sort of thing is happening the patient and practitioner are working together like dancing partners.

Here is an eminent practitioner and researcher making the point, with no concessions at all to the standard model of medical practice: '...acupuncture is not a theory, or even a collection of theories about disease and its treatment, but is an interpretative activity which involves the practitioner, the patient and the context' (MacPherson 1997, p.4).

I still remember the shock of reading that for the first time, not least because it seems to undercut so much of what I had struggled to learn and apply. But coming from someone of great experience and wisdom it demands careful consideration. It suggests, for one thing, that the decisions we make in the treatment room are not so much about the application of the principles of acupuncture to the complaints of the individual patient by the deductive process we were all taught, but are more to do with creating a coherent picture out of a combination of the patient's condition, his expectations of treatment, the practitioner's training, expertise and approach, and finally the context, which includes, as a minimum, any other treatment the patient is having and the circumstances of his life generally. The idea may become clearer with an example. An experienced teacher, happily married with two small children, stands in front of his class one day and freezes. He finds himself unable to talk. He opens his mouth but no words come out. Alarmed, he sees the boys and girls looking at him and their gaze is intolerable. Muttering some excuse he flees from the classroom. After a couple of minutes he is sufficiently composed to tell a colleague that he can't go back into the room and the children need to be supervised until the end of the lesson. Thereafter these panic attacks, as he calls them, start to recur with increasing frequency to the point where he is told to stay at home on sick leave for the rest of the term. His doctor prescribes anti-depressants, and he goes to see a counsellor. On the recommendation of a friend he also comes for acupuncture.

The TCM diagnosis might be Phlegm Fire Harassing the Heart, whereas a five element constitutional acupuncturist might have thought the main issue was a block between the Spleen and Heart channels. Palpation revealed a marked vacuity along the Pericardium and, to a lesser extent, the Liver channels. No doubt there were other diagnoses available, all consistent with traditional theories and all of which would suggest the points to be needled and in which order, and I am sure that a competent practitioner working along these lines would get reasonably good results. So where is the need for an 'interpretative activity', and what would it contribute to the treatment? Bearing in mind that his counsellor would be helping him to investigate and understand the reasons for this sudden change, what 'interpretative activity' is the province of the acupuncturist?

For one thing, it is unlikely that either the doctor or the counsellor would appreciate that it is his heart that has been deeply affected, and even if they did, they would know nothing of the pericardium and its role in what happened. They might not have been struck, either, by the fact that this capable man in his mid-forties arrived for treatment in shorts and a tee shirt on a day that was by no means warm. I expect they would have noticed that he was unwilling to make eye contact, and that when he did he wouldn't hold it for more than an instant, and also that he was oddly deferential for a man of his age and experience; but I suspect that they might not have been able to see the relevance of any of these things to his condition. And finally I imagine that both of them would have taken as read that the task was to restore the man to his former confidence in the classroom.

It all looks very different to an acupuncturist. Of course there will be a diagnosis and a series of treatments, but they will be founded on a view of this man's underlying energetic state, for which the observations above will provide crucial clues; on how the events that led up to his breakdown affected that state and brought it to the point of collapse; and lastly on what might be required to restore his strength and his resilience so that he can then do whatever he is called to, which might be to return to his previous job but it might not. The practitioner will bear in mind that his inability to stand in front of a classroom isn't necessarily a physical problem or even an emotional one, and from one perspective might not even be a problem at all but a cry from his spirit to do something different.

Naturally, the patient might not see it that way. And even if the practitioner comes to believe that this is indeed the case he will have to be sensitive to the fact that the patient may not see it as a possibility, may be resistant to such a view or may indeed reject it. The course of treatment will be a process of negotiation in which two people work together to come to a common view of what has happened and what would be the best outcome. At best it is a profoundly creative process, and it will take the practitioner far from the safe shores of textbook diagnoses and treatments. Certainly these provide an essential starting point, rather like the first buoy at the mouth of the harbour, but before long the practitioner will have to find his own way following intuitive instincts that have been honed by long experience.

Needling

Needling is the most basic thing we do in every treatment. Being habitual, it may seem straightforward, but it presents us with many puzzles. I was taught, for example, that there was a correct needle depth for each point, but then I had treatment from a Toya Hari practitioner who didn't insert the needle at all but held it a micro millimetre over the point above the skin. It hurt far more than any inserted needle had done and the results were excellent – so where are points exactly? And, after this experience, what depth should I go to when I insert? Even with the very best of teachers, Huang Di was confused about this:

> Huang Di asked, 'Could you please tell me about proper needling depth in acupuncture?'
>
> Qi Bo answered, 'When needling the bone level take care not to injure the tendon level. When needling the tendon level do not injure the muscles. When needling the muscles, do not injure the channels and vessels. When needling the channels, do not injure the skin...'
>
> Huang Di said, 'I do not feel I truly understand this.' (Ni 1995, p.186)

I know how he feels.

And how long should the needles stay in? In some traditions, tonification is with a quick insertion and removal, while in others the needles can be retained for twenty minutes or more. Here again is advice from Qi Bo:

> Observe the traveling of the qi with acupuncture in order to determine the best time to remove the needles. The arrival of qi, though not visible to the eye, is as if a flock of birds has converged. When the qi is leaving, it is as if the birds in a flock have scattered simultaneously. You cannot find a trace of them. Thus, when acupuncturing, if the qi has not arrived one should retain the needle as if one has drawn a bow in the ready position. As soon as the qi has arrived in the proper proportion, quickly remove the needle as if the arrow is being released. (Ni 1995, p.102)

Eloquent advice but not easy to follow. I could go on and on with these examples because there is a real difficulty, not just with needle depths and retention, but with any decision you make when needling, which is that you are relying on feeling specific sensations at the tip of the needle and then drawing inferences from them. In one way, it is a simple human ability, not so different from using a knife or a hammer. You start by feeling the tool in your hand but then, somehow, your awareness shifts to a sense of what is happening at the point where the knife cuts the onion or the hammer hits the nail. But this is enormously crude compared with the way a highly skilled acupuncturist gathers information from the tip of the needle as it seeks the Qi, touches and moves it – and all that in the blink of an eye. There's a lot going on.

> ...in order to stop the pathogen in its tracks, you must be patient and observant and wait for it to arrive. You insert the needle just before the pathogen arrives. This enables you to properly disperse. It is very intricate and delicate. If the needle is inserted too soon or too late, you will not

reach the pathogen; you will also injure the body. Mastery of acupuncture is like using a bow and arrow; you must know the precise moment to unleash the arrow. Mediocre acupuncturists are like those who hammer a wooden nail, dull and imprecise. You must find the right moment, and without hesitation, but with clarity, then you insert the needle. (Ni 1995, p.108)

The most important thing seems to be choosing exactly the right moment to insert the needle. This was never mentioned when I was at college – things are probably better now – where the assumption was that once you had found the point you just did it. A later workshop added the helpful notion of centring oneself and being stable before needling, but I've never heard anyone explain how to decide when is 'the precise moment' before the pathogen arrives.

Over the years I've looked for reliable indicators, wondering if they are different for the arrival of Damp Heat, for example, or Cold, but I've not been able to find any. However, the search has not been fruitless because it has taught me to be more aware of what is happening as I bend over a point, needle in hand. When I am ready I often pause, to see if there is anything that suggests I should wait: a tightness in the patient's muscles, which might relax, perhaps, with a little more pressure from my left hand; a sense of something gathering or being summoned, the way a tennis player calls up his power just before an explosive serve; an agitation in the patient that keeps his energy in a jumbled vortex up in his chest. The words hardly capture what is, in the moment, no more than a catch in the breath, a tiny impulse to stay the hand, which is as near as I can get to the notion of waiting for the pathogen to arrive. It is decision-making that is entirely intuitive.

It is the explanation too, I think, for those occasions when I think I have found the point under my fingertip, but when

I put the guide tube there it suddenly disappears – or at any rate, I find myself shifting the tube uneasily from the original location. I go a bit lateral or medial, a bit distal or proximal, change the angle of insertion, sometimes taking the tube off and feeling again with my finger. I fuss around the point like a dog that can't settle in its basket. I used to think it was because my point location measurements weren't accurate enough (from where on the elbow, precisely, do you measure cun to find points on the Sanjiao channel?), but now I think it is usually because the Qi hasn't arrived yet. So although I can find the point, there is nothing there, as yet, to needle.

I am sure that, like me, your needle technique has changed over the years and that the countless hours of practice have enhanced your intuitive knowledge of how the needle can respond more and more accurately to the patient's Qi. It is as if the repetition has stilled the thinking mind so that another kind of knowing can emerge. Recently I found the following quotation and was delighted to discover that something I had found myself doing instinctively is well known to musicians and chefs. It seems that those of us whose work requires highly precise manual skills all end up discovering the same truths.

> The idea of minimum force as the base line of self control is expressed in the apocryphal if perfectly logical advice given in ancient Chinese cooking; the good cook must learn first to cleave a grain of boiled rice... For physiological reasons that are not well understood, the ability to withdraw force in the microsecond after it is applied also makes the gesture itself more precise; one's aim improves. So in playing the piano, where the ability to release a key is an integral motion with pressing it down, finger pressure must cease at the moment of contact... In the musical hand, for this reason, it is harder to produce a clear soft sound than to belt out loud notes. (Sennett 2009, pp.167–8)

How many times have you identified the correct anatomical location of a point, but once you felt for it with your finger you knew that it wasn't exactly there? How many times have you angled your needle correctly to tonify, but found that somehow it needed to go in at a shallower, or more acute, angle? And how many times have you reached a perfectly plausible diagnosis but when you spelt out the points you would then have to do they didn't seem quite right? In all these instances you are experiencing the difference between the decisions you make with your rational mind and the promptings of your intuition. Through all of our education we were led to believe that the rational mind is more likely to be right, and it can be hard to recover from this bias. Of course, intuitive decisions are as prone to error as rational ones and we need to have some way of testing them before acting. And we can learn to enhance our natural intuitive abilities – both topics of later chapters. For now, all you need to accept is that you do in fact use your intuition all the time in the treatment room, that it is a legitimate way to make many of the decisions you face and that there are abundant benefits to be had from those moments when you just know – without knowing how it is you know. At the very least it may help you not to furrow your brow too deeply as you work.

CHAPTER 7

Cultivation

Although intuition is a natural ability it is more highly developed in some people than others. Perhaps the fortunate ones were born with it or maybe their circumstances lead them to learn to use it more than most, but anyone can cultivate it so that it grows and flourishes in them.

I have deliberately chosen to use a gardening metaphor. For one thing, as I will explain later, images and metaphors play a crucial role in evoking intuition. For another, just as with plants, you can't create it; all you can do is to help it grow – which doesn't sound much until you think of the difference between the crops of a skilled and experienced gardener and those of a novice, or indeed the stories of the penetrating insight of the masters of acupuncture.

> Bian Que, the legendary physician, says that although he knows four methods of assessment and the method of taking the pulse he does not bother with them... His art, it seems, is to discern the pattern instantaneously; he 'intuitively apprehended its general movement'. (Kaptchuk 2000, pp.288–9)

Good gardeners create the optimum conditions for their plants. The soil is weeded because weeds will take nutrients from them, and pests are removed because they will feed on the plants and weaken them; whatever might hinder their development is removed. Another strategy is to encourage and amplify growth by planting them in the right places, spreading manure and watering them. All of which applies to the cultivation of intuition. If you want to improve your own innate ability then you need to remove whatever is stunting it and then give it some nourishment instead – weeding and feeding.

I am sure we have all had moments when an intuition has arisen in us only to be instantly dismissed as ridiculous, foolish or fantastical. While not everything that comes to us in those moments is true or reliable, if we reject it all then we'll be throwing out the baby with the bathwater; nor will we ever learn to use it more and better. So the first essential step is not to suppress your intuitions. If you censor them immediately you'll never know what gifts they might contain.

And following closely on behind, the next step is not to judge or criticise them either; it'd be like spraying them with a toxin. What they are good at is indicating possibilities you hadn't thought of, grasping an entirety all at once and providing insight into the hidden nature of things. If your rational mind demands that you defend any of these intuitions by explaining exactly how you arrived at them and precisely why they are correct, then they may well fail the test. But it is simply the wrong test. In any case, just because you don't judge or criticise them doesn't mean you are going to act on every one of them. All you are doing is allowing them to survive, and then seeing if they can help.

I recently saw a patient for the second time and in the course of our conversation she started to talk about things she hadn't mentioned in the first session, things that had been very hard for her in the past. She paused, tears came into her eyes, and as they did she looked away from me and upwards to the left, into a corner of the room above the cupboard where I keep my acupuncture supplies. The first time she did this the thought came to me, 'It's as if the most important person in the room is sitting on top of the cupboard.' A ridiculous idea. I noticed it and carried on with the conversation, though the same thought occurred to me each time she did it. After the fourth time a silence fell; it seemed as if neither of us had any more to say. I waited for a few seconds, then asked, 'Is there someone on top of the cupboard?' It turned out there was.

Judgement or criticism of this intuition would have killed it. And significantly it arose when there was a pause in the conversation, for it seems that quiet of some kind is the soil in which intuition grows. Everyone who writes about it emphasises the need to quieten the mind: 'Intuitions come out of the silent mind' (Goldstein 1976, p.68); 'Activating intuition always starts with a shift into softness and silence' (Pierce, cited in Myers 2002, p.47); you need to 'learn to differentiate between internal noise and subtle incoming information that can only be perceived by silencing the mind' (Brennan 1988, p.9).

I know they are right. But saying I need to quieten my mind makes me think of those people who tell me to relax, as if it were something I could do by flicking a switch. In the treatment room I am busy trying to remember if Enid is the patient's sister or her mother, wondering if her voice has a weeping or groaning quality to it, thinking how to explain the energetics of multiple sclerosis or being frustrated that Liv 8 is so hard to locate – let alone trying to remember if I shut the upstairs window when it starts to rain – so there is indeed no space for any intuition to arise. How do I quiet the mind? If I ask it to stop it simply points to all the tasks that have to be done.

It helps to see intuition as arising from a strong Yin energy, from that deep interior stillness that in our culture we sometimes call the unconscious, so that instead of asking how to quiet the mind we can think of allowing our Yin energy to predominate for a while. I put down my pen, relax my shoulders, feel my body getting heavier in the chair; I take a few deeper breaths in my lower abdomen and sit still as I listen to the patient, and each time I think of something to say I let it go without giving it another moment's thought.

It is especially easy to amplify my Yin energy when the patient is on the couch. After I have taken the pulses and looked at the tongue I often say I'm going to take a minute or two to think about the treatment, so there will be a bit of a pause before I start to needle. That gives me the opportunity to sit still in my chair or to stand at the window and gaze out (there's a wonderful view). I don't try to think coherently; I just get still and wait and see what comes to me. In a way it is the opposite of how we expect intuition to work; we assume, I think, that it is a kind of jumping to conclusions, whereas in fact it arises from pausing, waiting and allowing.

This 'allowing' has a noble lineage, for it is in the great tradition of wu wei. Applied to thinking it is Yin, whereas logic and reasoning are Yang.

> Wu Wei...must be understood primarily as a form of intelligence – that is, of knowing the principles, structures and trends of human and natural affairs so well that one uses the least amount of energy in dealing with them. But this intelligence...is not simply intellectual; it is also the 'unconscious' intelligence of the whole organism. (Watts 1992, p.76)

That minute or two of quiet is an opportunity for a deeper truth to be revealed. For one thing, I think the silence serves to increase my sensitivity so that I am more likely to pick up some resonance from the patient, some unspoken message that might lead me to a more accurate treatment. And it also gives me a chance to notice how I am feeling.

The body often knows before the mind. In a famous experiment, gamblers were given two decks of cards – one red, one blue – and were asked to turn over one card at a time from whichever deck they wanted. They were also told that each card would bring them a financial gain or loss. The decks were stacked. The red one gave some handsome rewards but also some big penalties, and in the end the more cards you turned over the more you would lose. The blue one gave only modest rewards and penalties, but in the long run yielded a profit. The idea was to see how long it took the gamblers to work out which deck to use, and also to see if this matched the reading from sensors that picked up the activity of sweat glands in the hands.

> ...gamblers started generating stress responses to the red decks by the tenth card, forty cards before they were able to say they had a hunch about what was wrong with those two decks. More important, right around the time their palms started sweating, their behavior began to change as well. They started favoring the blue cards and taking fewer and fewer cards from the red deck. In other words, the gamblers figured the game out before they realized they had figured the game out: they began making the necessary adjustments long before they were consciously aware of what adjustments they were supposed to be making. (Gladwell 2005, pp.9–10)

If only my mind knew what my body has already grasped! Perhaps while the cogs of my brain are still grinding, my body has already reached a diagnosis, made a treatment plan and chosen points. Although I might not be able to tap into its decision-making process, I can at least be alert to signs that it has been working and has something to say. Suddenly feeling cold or tired, sensing a disturbance in my left lower abdomen (quite a common indicator for me) or tightening my lower lip are all signs to me that I'm experiencing something that I haven't realised I've noticed. Some of these signs can be tiny and fleeting, so unless your mind is quiet you may well miss them.

> Intuition on the emotional level can function fully only when you are aware of feelings, without judging them as good or bad and without assuming you have to act on them or do anything about them. There is no need to justify or rationalise a feeling... It is not possible to genuinely get into your work or be open to intimacy if you are out of touch with your feelings. (Vaughan 1979, pp.26–7)

There is one last benefit to the quietness, which is that it gets me out of the mindset (as if I didn't know better) of doing exactly the right treatment that will immediately improve my patient's symptoms. Of course I want to work well and of course I want my patients to get better, but having those goals in my mind distorts what I can see and hear and feel, and leads me away from the work that the patient really needs me to do. In other words, as so many masters of acupuncture have said, the best work happens when the practitioner gets out of the way, and moments of silence allow this to happen.

Play

So far I have been talking about the conditions that favour intuition; now I want to turn to how it can be encouraged. You can't force it and you certainly can't make it happen by an act of will, but there are some things that can trigger it; and if you do them then a moment of insight often follows. I'm going to describe a few different triggers but they have in common a quality of playfulness. Here is Valerie Hunt describing how she made a fundamental breakthrough:

> Timidly I placed the electromyographic (EMG) recording electrodes on her lower arm, her upper arm and her back muscles, each area primarily stimulated by a different level of the spinal cord and brain. Intuitively, in a playful mood, I placed one electrode on top of her head, although I knew nothing about chakras... At the beginning nothing unusual happened... Yet, in five minutes the recordings remarkably changed. The muscular signal from her lower arm stopped. The baseline activity characteristic of all living tissue was absent on the scopes. Next, the lower arm recordings dropped out. The engineer believed there was no equipment failure... Next, electromagnetic energy poured from the top of her head with intensity beyond what our equipment could handle... In my years of neuromuscular research I had never witnessed any similar situation, nor had any been described in the literature. (Hunt 1996, pp.10–11)

She had no reason to put that last electrode on top of the head, but without it she would have missed a crucial lesson from the experiment. The 'playful mood' comes from doing something that makes no sense to the rational mind and hence seems completely pointless – but it might still be exactly and precisely what is needed. Because we often treat people who are in pain or distress, or coping with some dysfunction or disability, we might tend to squash the impulse to do something playful; it might seem irreverent. But that may be to ignore the prompting of our own unconscious wisdom.

Jonas Salk, the chemist who created the polio vaccine, had no difficulty in allowing an active imagination to stimulate his rigorous research:

> When I became a scientist, I would picture myself as a virus or as a cancer cell, for example, and try to sense what it would be like to be either. I would also imagine myself as the immune system, and I would try to reconstruct what I would do as an immune system engaged in combating

a virus or cancer cell. When I had played through a series
of such scenarios on a particular problem I would design
laboratory experiments accordingly. (Salk 1983, p.7)

What he is doing is to separate two modes of thinking. He first
allows his creativity full rein and only later does he bring his
rational intellect to bear on what it has produced. In this way
he encourages his intuitive mind to work and protects it from
interference by logic.

> Intuition...does feel like a dream or a memory in the sense
> that intuitive sensations are very delicate and, as with a
> dream, the slightest external disturbance can turn the
> dream or the intuitive impression into a fog. (Shealey and
> Myss 1988, p.85)

All this suggests that we need to find a way of stimulating our
own creativity in the treatment room. There are many well-
known techniques and I want to describe three of them that
I have found helpful and easy to use. The first is to look for
images and metaphors.

A metaphor works by comparing two things that are not
at all similar – as at the start of this chapter where I compared
cultivating plants to cultivating intuition. Forcing these two
very different things together leads you to think of similarities
that you would never have imagined otherwise, and that sparks
novel ideas. It is that spark, I think, that fires our intuition.

I got quite frustrated with one patient who was overweight,
who never seemed able to change her eating habits and who
wasn't doing at all well with treatment. One day I looked for an
image that might help and suddenly saw her as a galleon under
full sail (it had to be a galleon; to call her 'a large sailing ship'
would not capture the essence of the woman), and I realised
that for that galleon to change course and turn around would
take the work of a lot of skilled hands. It is so interesting how

a metaphor brings along its own language with it; 'hands' is such a suggestive pun. So I said that instead of seeing me each week she should have regular treatments with one of each of the following: a cranial osteopath, a Rolfer, a herbalist and me. Getting all of them on board (another pun) made all the difference; it took the pressure off me, so I worked better, and having a variety of treatments really suited her.

Another example is of a young woman who enjoyed her treatments and they helped with various minor complaints, but I couldn't help feeling that I only got occasional glimpses of who she really was, certainly not enough to feel confident in my work and to really understand what she needed. Taking her pulses one day I looked at her face and caught her unawares. She met my gaze for a split second, then quickly turned away. And I remembered paddling in the sea one day and seeing a flash of silver as a small fish turned and dashed away from my foot. In an instant she was that fish. And I realised for the first time how huge and powerful and lumbering I was to her, and how she was frightened of me as she had been frightened of so many people in her life. From then on I had a much better idea of how to work with her.

When patients use images or metaphors they can often trigger intuition just as much as when you use them yourself. A very anxious woman who had been persistently unwell for some time told me that it was all because of a complex set of emotional problems, which she referred to as 'a ball of wax'. It was such an unusual and vivid image that I knew immediately it was telling me something. (Because she was Canadian I thought I'd better check that it did indeed have a personal meaning, so I asked her if that was a cliché or common phrase in her country; she told me it wasn't.) It seemed to me that it might help her to resolve these problems and relieve her anxiety if the wax was melted. After all, she wasn't saying it was a ball of concrete or manure or impossibly tangled string, but that it could be dissolved. I did mainly Fire points and used a lot of moxa.

When I get the feeling that there is something I haven't quite thought of saying to the patient, or that there is some question I haven't managed to formulate, or maybe even that something has been left unsaid between us that needs to be acknowledged, I use a different trigger. I announce that I have something to say although I have absolutely nothing in mind. I got the idea from a poem:

> As a queen sits down, knowing that a chair will be there,
> Or a general raises his hand and is given the field glasses,
> Step off assuredly into the blank of your mind.
> Something will come to you.

(Wilbur 2004, p.54)

If queens and generals, why not acupuncturists? So I pause for a moment to give my intuition time to put into words what I only know as the vaguest of feelings, then I open my mouth and the words come out. I listen to them with interest, for they are as much news to me as they are to my patient. They usually strike me as perfectly sensible, but quite often they are better than that. They answer some question the patient hasn't had the courage to ask, for example, or touch some vulnerable place with reassuring kindness. Whatever they do specifically, they always seem to bring more intimacy into the relationship. I don't really know why this is so, but I do think that we pick up far more information than we are conscious of and I suspect that our underlying desire to help our patients then puts that information to good use.

At the end of a treatment, after all the needles are out, I often find there is something I want to say. I may have come to some understanding of the patient's condition – sudden hair loss is one recent instance – and I think it would help the patient to know why it has happened; or I have a suggestion for what the patient can do to manage a condition better; or I need to revise the timing and frequency of treatments. So I tell the patient that when she is off the couch and dressed I will have two (or three) things to say – when actually I only have one (or two) in mind. It is a simple variant of the same technique, but it feels less risky. For one thing, your intuition has a bit longer to come up with the goods, and for another, if it fails to do so the patient probably won't notice that you are one thing short. And again I usually find myself saying something helpful.

The last trigger for stimulating intuition is good for those times when I feel bogged down with a patient. Either I am not managing the relationship well or I simply can't see the appropriate diagnosis or I don't understand why the patient's energy system reacts to treatment in the way it does. Essentially it is because I'm stuck in a particular way of thinking. Most of the time these thinking habits work well, but when they don't, they don't work at all. It isn't practical to try and change them, but it is possible to short circuit them. That's an image from electricity. Sparks fly when an abnormal connection is made as it delivers a large amount of energy in a short space of time. Ideal for our purposes.

Assume for a moment that when we think through what to do with a patient we follow a habitual circuit, which goes like this:

> T.C.M. is a rational style of medicine which follows a step by step progression from information collected by the four examinations to the statement of treatment principles and thence to the erection of a treatment plan based on those principles. (Flaws 1997, pp.112–13)

And he could have gone on to add further consequent stages, such as deciding what we need to treat first and what can wait until later, which points to select, what needle technique to use and so on. The logic means that we will always start in the same place and follow the same sequence. But if we want to short circuit the process then we need to start somewhere different. We can pick anywhere in the process; it doesn't matter where because the idea is simply to jolt us out of our habits.

So, for example, the next time one of these patients comes for treatment you might simply walk up to the couch and see which point you are drawn to needle; you don't have to actually do it, but you look to see if there is any rationale for that point that might lead you to a new view of the patient and a new diagnosis. When you do this you might find yourself smiling, almost laughing out loud. It often has that flavour of a joke, for that too depends on making some new and unexpected mental connection. Once again, there is so often something light-hearted about intuition.

A more radical version of the same technique is to start your thinking with anything that catches your attention, even if it seems completely irrelevant. The sun may come out and cast a shadow across the patient's chest; you might happen to glance at her left shoe as she takes it off and notice that the heel is badly worn on one side; or, for no apparent reason, you find yourself humming a tune you haven't heard for years. These three examples are different in many ways, but what they have in common is that they present opportunities for your intuition to speak. They are good new starting places. Perhaps in the first example the lungs need treating, or in the second there is an imbalance between the left and right sides of the patient's body, or finally there are words in the song that sum up the situation precisely. It is a long way away from accepted practice, but that is precisely the point.

Ritual

There is one last thing to say about the whole business of cultivating your intuitive skills and powers. As with any skill it improves with practice and withers if left unused, so even if you feel hesitant about relying on your intuition, which is sensible if you are inexperienced, you can still practise it with each patient. You can create a moment or two of quiet, you can ask yourself if an image suggests itself, you can pay attention first to the patient's spirit rather than her symptoms, and in all these instances take note of any insights that come to you. You don't have to act on them; you may choose for a while simply to reflect on them. If you notice that you are getting more and more accurate then you can start to use them with confidence.

If you want to amplify the power of this practice then it is a good idea to turn it into a kind of ritual. The monk who chants the Heart Sutra for the umpteenth time and the Catholic priest who blesses the wine and water each week both know that repetition deepens their understanding.

There is no need for us to follow a prescribed ritual; we can each devise our own. Mine, for what it is worth, is to take a moment or two of quiet just after I pick up the patient's hand to take the pulses for the first time in the session; I think that I pick up information from simply being in touch with the patient before my mind gets busy with pulse strengths and qualities. I then take another moment or two of quiet after I pick up the first needle; I think that pause is to give my intuition a chance to come up with a better idea. From time to time I do all the other things I have described in this chapter, but these are my rituals and I do them every time. They are some of my happiest times in the treatment room, for what can make a practitioner happier than suddenly knowing exactly what would best serve the patient that day?

CHAPTER 8

Reliability

There are those who are sceptical of intuition. Some say that there is really no such thing and that people who claim to be intuitive are either just guessing or simply thinking so quickly that it looks like an intuitive leap. Then there are others who point out that when experts use their intuition they very often make mistakes. So the Nobel Prize winner Daniel Kahneman and his colleague Gary Klein asked the wonderful question: 'When can you trust an experienced professional who claims to have an intuition?' The results of their researches are of direct relevance to what we do in the treatment room, because we need to know if our own intuitions can be trusted.

The answer to their question starts with work done by a social psychologist who wondered if predictions made on the basis of a few simple rules and scores would be more accurate than those made by experts. For example, he got teachers to predict the grades that their students would get at the end of the year. Each student was given a forty-five-minute interview and the teachers also took into account the student's personal statement and his previous exam grades. The researcher then fed some very basic information about each student into an algorithm, and found that it yielded a different set of predictions. At the end of the year, when all the students' grades were known, he compared their results with the two predictions, and found that the algorithm was more accurate than the teachers. Somewhat surprised by this outcome, he repeated his research with a wide range of other professionals.

> Meehl reported generally similar results across a variety of other forecast outcomes, including violations of parole, success in pilot training and criminal recidivism... The range of predicted outcomes has been expanded to cover medical variables such as the longevity of cancer patients, the length of hospital stays, the diagnosis of cardiac disease, and the susceptibility of babies to sudden infant death syndrome... In every case the accuracy of experts was matched or exceeded by a simple algorithm. (Kahneman 2012, pp.222–3)

This is quite a challenge to us all. Does any one of us really believe that we would reach more accurate diagnoses if we keyed a few variables into our laptop or tablet and got an instant answer back? I doubt it. On the other hand, the evidence is unmistakable.

Rather charmingly, Kahneman tells how he caught himself believing in his own expertise. Over a considerable period of time he used various tests and interviews to assess the suitability of candidates for officer training in the army. He describes the powerful sense of getting to know each candidate and his intuitive conviction that as a result he could tell which person would do well as an officer and in combat. However:

> The evidence that we could not forecast success accurately was overwhelming... The dismal truth about the quality of our predictions had no effect whatsoever on how we evaluated candidates and very little effect on the confidence we felt in our judgments and predictions about individuals... The global evidence of our previous failure should have shaken our confidence in our judgments of candidates but it did not. (Kahneman 2012, p.211)

It made me wonder if I have a similarly misplaced confidence in my own judgement in the treatment room. Have I fallen into the same trap? Am I so confident of my intuition that I too ignore my failures and, even worse, write a book advocating it as a basis for acupuncture treatments?

Conditions

According to Kahneman and Klein, intuitions can be considered reliable if two conditions are met. The first is that the professional must work in what they call an orderly environment; that is one where the subject matter isn't prone to sudden and unpredictable change. So at one end of the scale, chess is highly orderly and the intuition of an expert chess player is to be trusted, while at the other end of the scale no one can reliably predict the movement of the stock market or events in a war. In their view medical practice is relatively orderly, for although human beings are astonishingly complex there are the regularities of bodily functions and disorders, so it does provide the opportunity to learn from repeated treatments. Although they say nothing about acupuncture I think Kahneman and Klein would regard it as a pretty orderly environment. We do see the same kinds of conditions over and over again and the people we treat usually come to us for a number of sessions. Although one person's asthma may be very different from another's, there are regularities such as the distinction between struggling to breathe in and struggling to breathe out, or the common link between asthma and eczema. And, most crucially, Qi in the human body flows in orderly ways, for the meridian charts in every textbook are all the same, as are (almost all) point locations. There are classic descriptions too of the way Qi typically becomes depleted, stagnates or sinks.

The second condition for reliability is that people need to be able to learn from their mistakes, so prolonged practice and good feedback are both essential. Learning to drive a car is relatively easy because each time the novice driver gets the balance between clutch and accelerator wrong the car either bounds off down the road in kangaroo leaps or it stalls and stops dead. The feedback is instant and unequivocal.

The importance of feedback is highlighted when comparing two kinds of medical professionals. 'Experienced radiologists who evaluate chest X rays as "normal" or "abnormal" contradict themselves 20% of the time when they see the same picture on separate occasions' (Kahneman 2012, p.225). There are good reasons for this rather startling statistic:

> Among medical specialities, anesthesiologists benefit from good feedback because the effects of their actions are likely to be quickly evident. In contrast, radiologists obtain little information about the accuracy of the diagnoses they make and about the pathologies they fail to detect. Anesthesiologists are therefore in a better position to develop useful intuitive skills. If an anesthesiologist says 'I have a feeling something is wrong,' everyone in the operating room should be prepared for an emergency. (Kahneman 2012, p.242)

We have the opportunity to get plenty of feedback. In my opinion, the pulses never fail to tell me if I have chosen the right point or points. Yesterday, I treated a new patient whose balance has been poor since he had a stroke three years ago and who now has difficulty walking without a stick. I made my diagnosis and set about treating him. After needling the first point I took his pulses and there was absolutely no change in them at all. I thought his system might be a bit sluggish so I decided to persist with the diagnosis. I needled the point I had planned to do next and got the same result. So I refined my diagnosis and did two more points accordingly – with exactly the same result. I ended up with one last idea, and one last point, and that made not the slightest difference either. I usually do better. But at least I got immediate and unmistakable feedback, and I did learn something.

Patients also give us feedback when they tell us how they have been since the previous treatment. I can't overstate the importance of this. One patient came to me because she had suffered from headaches for the previous twenty years. I encouraged her to keep records of how she was each day so she could see if there were any clues as to what might be triggering them and also help her to assess if treatment was helping. She took to the task with great enthusiasm and within a few weeks discovered that she actually had three different types of headaches and that one of them, oddly, was accompanied by a small sharp pain in a toe on her left foot. A few more weeks passed and she became aware that each headache had a different cause. A few more weeks and she found she could avoid two kinds of headaches by spotting danger signs and managing the conditions that brought them on. That left one kind of headache for me to deal with, and by then a diagnosis was quite clear. I am quite certain that if she had not done this work and I had tried to treat three different kinds of headaches at once, without even knowing they were different, I would not have been able to help.

By contrast, there are those patients who, when asked how they have been since the last time, respond by saying things like, 'Oh, much the same,' or 'Maybe a bit better,' or 'I had a good day on Thursday, or was it Friday? Actually, it might have been the week before.' I just can't learn enough from them to have confidence in my diagnosis or treatment plan, let alone any intuitive ideas about what they might need. It is of course my responsibility to explain why good feedback is crucial to the treatment process and to help them learn to pay closer attention to themselves, so I now insist that they keep at least a brief daily record of any changes, especially surprising ones.

You can sometimes get feedback from patients during a treatment. I have a few who comment on how they feel after a particular point, and it is always illuminating. And every now and then there are some exceptional opportunities to learn.

There's a woman I've been treating for about fifteen years. She was trained as a five element constitutional acupuncturist and likes to be treated with mainly Wood points. In a recent session I asked her, 'What would you like today?' I often do this with her because she likes to be asked, even if she sometimes doesn't know or prefers to leave it to me. She replied straight away, 'Balance.' Alright, I thought, that's a nice clear goal. As we talked a little more, and as I looked at her tongue and took her pulses, I found myself thinking of Metal points. When I paused to wonder why they kept occurring to me I thought they might restrain what seemed to me that day to be a rather excessive ebullience, a kind of forced determination to make changes in her life with vim and vigour. And when she had talked about these changes I couldn't help noticing that I wasn't completely convinced.

So I said to her, 'I'm considering Metal points.' She pulled her knees up to her chest, wrapped her hands around them and rocked to and fro on the couch. She went bright red in the face and said, 'Ohhh. Ohhh, I don't know about that.'

Seeing I was a little surprised at her reaction she gave me a number of reasons why she was alarmed at the prospect, and after hearing them I was quite willing to abandon the idea. I spent quite a while trying to come up with a sensible alternative treatment, so long in fact that she had time to reconsider. 'Go on then,' she said. 'It's alright.' So I did Metal points.

The next day, somewhat anxiously, I waited for her report. She emailed saying the treatment had been great, that she had felt much calmer than for a long time and that it was a relief to have her Wood energy in check for once. 'After all,' she wrote, 'Metal does control Wood on the Ke cycle.'

It was a good opportunity to test my intuition, for this patient felt able to alert me to the risks of giving her an unusual treatment and she could also give me quick, precise feedback on it too. These times, and they do happen now and again, present us with golden opportunities.

More generally, if you want to improve the reliability of your intuition you need to get feedback each time you use it; and in order to do that you have to keep some kind of record of what happened. It is not just a matter of looking at your notes to see if the patient responded well to the treatment – that won't be nearly specific enough. For one thing, the intuition will have opened up new ways of thinking about your patient's energy and how best to treat it – in the example above it showed me that tonifying her Wood, which is what she expects from treatment, may not be what she really needs, or at least not always.

There are many other possibilities too. For example, your intuition might tell you one day, somewhat to your surprise, that a treatment was complete after only one or two points, so you'll need to know if your patient's response was different from after previous treatments. Or intuition might have something to say about the relationship between the two of you. Perhaps your instinct one day was to challenge a patient for the first time, pointing out, for instance, that if she wants to lose weight she simply has to take more exercise and eat healthier food. You will need to note what effect that had on her, on the treatment you chose to do and on how you related to each other afterwards.

And then there is the need to record how confident you were when you used your intuition. If, looking back, you find that when you are not very confident then it doesn't work out well, but that the outcome is wonderful when you are, then you will have a clear guide for the future. And if you were to find that your supreme confidence is routinely misplaced then, well, it might be best to give it up and stick to the tried and tested.

Signs

It turns out that experienced and busy acupuncturists will be able to meet the challenge posed by Kahneman and Klein and can have a great deal of confidence in their intuitions. But their research only reaches general conclusions and doesn't answer the nagging question that comes up over and over again in the treatment room. That is: Can I trust this particular intuition with this particular patient? In other words, is there a way of distinguishing, in the moment, between random hunches and genuine intuitions?

With unconscious inferences there is the option of jogging backwards to see if the instant intuition could also have been arrived at by the sequential steps of analytical reasoning. If so then it is trustworthy; indeed it is no more than a speedy application of the normal principles of Chinese medicine. But you may not have time for that, and in any case this test won't work with the kinds of intuition I have called hints and whispers or sudden knowings. Something else is needed.

Thoughts run through our minds all the time during the course of any treatment. Most of them are fleeting, some may be interesting and a few can lead to a useful conclusion, but they all lack the power and potential of intuitions. The difference between a hunch and a genuine intuition isn't always obvious, so it is helpful to know that there are some reliable signs of intuition at work.

In general, what marks out genuine intuitions is a quality of truthfulness. They seem to reveal something about the patient that the practitioner hadn't seen before, and that, once seen, is not doubted; or they may suddenly bring to mind the precise point or point combination that will best treat that person at that particular stage of his healing. They may even reveal something about the practitioner, showing why one patient isn't getting better, or why another who seemed to be doing well has stopped coming.

One specific sign of genuine intuition that is especially useful when you are worried about a patient or lack confidence in your diagnosis is when an idea brings an immediate feeling of calm. A deeply knowledgeable practitioner, one who is steeped in the classics, told me that when his intuition, as opposed to his reasoning, comes up with an answer, 'My system relaxes. The decision's been made and it's out of my hands.' It is a striking phrase, echoed by other practitioners I have talked to about this. In one way or another they all recognise this feeling of relief, almost as if the treatment is no longer up to them any more but comes from the power of the intuition itself. And for a number of them the calm is not just in them but affects everything at once, so the atmosphere in the room gets quieter, lighter and gentler too. One practitioner, musing upon this phenomenon, saw it as the experience of balance. When, even if only for a moment, Yin and Yang are held together in perfect symmetry, she told me, then unity appears; and it is from that deeper reality that unimagined possibilities arise.

Another sign is when an idea arrives accompanied by an unshakeable conviction. Once a genuine intuition has occurred to you then you may want to think about its rationale and the way it expresses or exemplifies some aspect of Chinese medicine, but you don't doubt it and you don't wonder if it might be worth thinking again. It is impossible to confuse this with thoughts of the kind, 'I wonder if...' or 'Maybe I should...' or 'I could try...' What has come to you is a complete and perfect answer to the question you have been asking, so it would be ridiculous to go on looking. It has the quality of a wish being granted; there is that element of magic about receiving exactly what you asked for.

One practitioner gave me a wonderful example. A patient arrived for treatment complaining that for three and a half weeks out of four she was not herself, that she was 'snappy, vile and actively unpleasant to my long-suffering husband'. On questioning her it seemed that it had all started about nine months previously, after she had her gall bladder removed. Her pulses were good, if a little rapid, and her tongue was good too, if a little red around the edges. The practitioner toyed with clearing Heat or dispersing Liver, but then had the idea of needling GB 41 and TB 5. In that moment, as he said, 'It was the only thing I could possibly do as a treatment.' The patient came back saying that she had stopped being so unpleasant and indeed that she had stopped some extreme behaviours that she had not told him about before.

Another common sign is when the idea comes as a complete surprise. Not only was there no inkling of it before it arrived, but also even in retrospect it is hard to see that it could have come from any normal thinking process. It can, for example, lead you to an area of the body you would not otherwise have considered. A successful professional athlete came for treatment because her career was threatened by a recurrent ankle injury, and she had tried everything else without success. Her practitioner examined the ankle carefully and then, for reasons he cannot explain, went straight to GB 31 where he did some Tui Na. He then needled GB 40 followed by SJ 5 on the opposite side. She resumed training the next day. Anyone might think of needling these two points (though they are only one of many possible options), but he is certain that they would have had little effect if he had not first opened up the tissue at GB 31.

Another practitioner often hears herself asking a question or making a comment that comes as a surprise. She gave me the example of a soft and gentle woman, endlessly patient and compassionate, who had endured the deaths of her parents and husband, all from cancer and all in the space of a year. The poor woman managed to recover from this triple blow and a few years later found happiness again and remarried. Shortly after returning from her honeymoon, her new husband was diagnosed with cancer. Her practitioner, when told the news, simply had no words. What could she possibly say? Then her mouth opened and she found herself shouting, 'You must be *furious*!' At that moment everything changed. The patient raged and said things she had expressed to no one and had not admitted to herself. And for the first time the practitioner saw who she really was and felt that for the first time she really knew how best to treat her.

Another useful sign comes from your own feelings. The arrival of an intuition feels quite different from following a train of thought and working out the possible interactions between the various syndromes. The former is more like an experience, such as knowing you are too hot or whether you are attracted to the person you have just met. Indeed, the arrival of an intuition is often accompanied by a body-felt sensation. Here are some examples from fellow practitioners with whom I have discussed this: one told me, 'my mouth fills with saliva'; another said, 'I get a tingling sensation in my hands'; a third added, 'my heart starts to beat faster'; and finally one I recognise myself, 'excitement runs through my body'. Barbara Hepworth, the famous artist and sculptor, said, 'I rarely draw what I see – I draw what I feel in my body' (Hepworth, cited in Smith 2014, p.4). It is a remarkable thing to say; it seems impossible, but I think she is saying exactly what it is like when you allow intuition to guide your work.

Finally in a chapter that has been concerned with questioning the reliability of intuition, I want to close with an inspiring story of someone who uses his intuition in moments of acute danger and has found it wholly dependable:

> There's this guy up on the roof, right at the edge, with his infant son in his arms; he's threatening to throw him off and then jump himself. Homicide – suicide – happens a lot with children. He's been having trouble with his wife ...he's sleeping in the hallway and it's gone to the edge. That's where he is and I'm up there with him. I'm the final guy in the hostage recovery system we set up in New York City, which I've been working in for eight years and heading up for the last two. We haven't lost anybody in all that time... Funny thing is I can't remember much of what I've been saying to people at the end of these episodes. I'm running very much on intuition from moment to moment. (Dass and Gorman 1986, pp.105, 107)

CHAPTER 9

Healing

We don't often need to question the fundamentals. It is usually pretty obvious what the patient wants, what we need to do in order to help and how to tell whether or not we are doing good work, so our normal ways of thinking about these things are perfectly adequate. But sometimes our routine approaches simply can't do justice to the complexity we encounter, and we are called to work at a deeper level. At these times even the most analytical of practitioners may find it essential to call on their intuition.

A patient comes to you with back pain. No doubt you have treated it many times before and know all the syndromes, but in the following example none of that would really help:

> In the first months of my practice a patient came to the clinic, grey and bent and with the pain of a terrible backache. He was a priest... Being in those days eager to 'make people well'...I can tell you that had I known how to treat his back symptomatically I would have done so. One day I entered the treatment room and saw him sitting fully dressed in the corner. My heart sank; 'He's come to tell me he's stopping treatment,' I thought, and yet, with curiosity, I noticed he was looking wonderful, radiant even. Sure enough, he said, 'Meriel, I have come to tell you I am stopping treatment but I want you to know that acupuncture has cured me. I didn't

tell you when I came for treatment of my greatest grief...
I didn't tell you that in recent years I had lost God, lost the
ability to pray, and have lived in such pain... Last night I
dreamed that God was speaking to me. He said, "Don't be
concerned about your back, I am with you." My back feels
fine today.' (Darby 2003, p.34)

If you had been the priest's practitioner do you think you would
have been able to perceive the real cause of his back pain, and
hence what he really needed from treatment? It's hard to see
how you could have reached such a diagnosis by any rational
means; surely only an intuitive leap could get you there. And
although his acupuncturist doesn't say so, she must have seen it
and treated it, even if she never articulated it clearly to herself.

It is sometimes quite a challenge to understand exactly
what a patient really wants from treatment and wants from
us. In a mild form this happens all the time; the complaint or
condition the patient first brings to us may well be only the
most superficial level of her illness, and as treatment proceeds
we often find ourselves tackling something very different. But
still, we usually assume that it is good to start by alleviating
the symptoms that are presented to us at the beginning. John
Updike would disagree:

...was not my sly strength, my insistent specialness, somehow
linked to my psoriasis? Might it not be the horrible badge
of whatever in me was worth honoring? ... Only psoriasis
could have taken a very average little boy, and furthermore
a boy who loved the average, the daily, the safely hidden,
and made him into a prolific, adaptable, ruthless-enough
writer. What was my creativity, my relentless need to
produce but a parody of my skin's overproduction? Was
not my thick literary skin which shrugged off rejection
slips and patronising reviews by the sheaf, a superior version
of my poor vulnerable own? ... And with my changeable

epiderm came a certain transcendent optimism; like a snake
I shed many skins... To my body...psoriasis is normal and
its suppression abnormal. Psoriasis is my health. (Updike
1990, pp.70–2)

Admittedly this is an extreme and exceptional example, but still,
as with the priest, the relief of symptoms is not necessarily what
our patients really need or want, even though they may not
know it or may only be able to express it in the most awkward of
ways. Many people in this culture lack the language to describe
spiritual distress and may struggle to express chronic feelings
of anxiety, worthlessness and so on. In these deep waters the
rational methods of diagnosis and treatment look inadequate,
and we may have to rely on our intuition to tell us that all is
not as it seems with a particular patient. The fundamental point
is as old as acupuncture itself. To repeat the famous words, 'In
order to make all acupuncture thorough and effective one must
first cure the spirit' (Veith 2002, pp.215–16).

It is so easy for busy practitioners to pay lip service to this
and still carry on treating bad knees, irritable bowels and
irregular periods as if the spirit was irrelevant. But it is good
to be reminded once again of 'the mysterious truth that the
spirit is the life of the body seen from within, and the body the
outward manifestation of the spirit – the two being really one'
(Jung 1985, p.253).

We all know that this system of medicine is intrinsically
holistic, and that needling a point will have an effect on the
person as a whole – what we conventionally call body, mind and
spirit – but Qi Bo and Jung (quite a combination) instruct us to
be more specific. They instruct us to pay attention to the spirit
precisely in order to treat a painful knee, a disturbed bowel
or a stagnant uterus. It works the other way round too; these
same symptoms can give us information about the state of the

patient's spirit, and we may come to treat it through reading the body's distress.

It isn't easy to do this. It is so much simpler to diagnose a patient with Blood deficiency, Liver Qi Stagnation or as a Wood constitutional type than to perceive a disturbance of spirit. Here is Qi Bo again telling us how to do it:

> The Shen can be observed through the patient's eyes. But the true vision is through your own eyes. What you receive as messages, your heart will understand. You can then visualise the patient's condition in your mind. You can intuitively know what the problem is. (Ni 1995, p.105)

In short, we sometimes need to use our intuition to tell us the true nature of our patient's illness. How do we read her body through her spirit and vice versa? And when are her symptoms part of her health, needing to be respected rather than confronted?

The same kind of thing is true of what we call psychosomatic illness, which is often taken to mean merely that people are more likely to succumb to viruses or bacteria after some emotional trauma, but there's much more to it than that. Here is a cancer surgeon: 'Years of experience have taught me that cancer and indeed nearly all diseases are psychosomatic. This may sound strange to people accustomed to thinking that psychosomatic ailments are not truly "real" but, believe me, they are' (Siegel 1986, p.111). And here is a remarkable passage from a man who devoted his life to relieving pain and improving function through working with his hands and whose teachings have spread all over the world:

> What I have learned is that no amount of physical treatment or manipulation can take away this back pain when I have it. But I can sit down in a quiet place and introspect about

whether I am angry or not, and if so, what about. When
I find the anger and resolve it my back pain automatically
goes away... Now I realise that when I am aware of being
angry my back doesn't hurt. It only hurts when I am angry
and don't know it. (Upledger 1997, pp.115–16)

If we were to have patients whose back (or bowel or head)
only hurts when they are angry, but who lack the skill of
introspection to realise it, then how do we treat them? And if
our treatment didn't work, and Dr Upledger is clear that in his
case no treatment would have worked, then how would we even
know why?

Qi

To some extent the answer to these kinds of awkward questions
lies in the wonder of Qi. We all know that when we treat Qi the
most extraordinary things can happen. People are touched at a
deep level and as a result may tell us something they didn't know
themselves until they said it; or a patient may feel refreshed,
enlivened and enriched by a treatment even though there is
no improvement in her symptoms; or, a final example from
my own practice, a treatment of a sixty-year-old patient's hip
problem made not much difference to the hip but resolved a
shoulder problem she had had since she was injured by a bomb
blast as a child. It is obvious, but still seems miraculous, how
touching Qi can have such profound and unpredictable effects.

But part of the answer to these questions must also lie in the
way we choose to work with a patient. A doctor writes: 'Healing
is not just a property of the physical body...healing, like health
and illness, must also be psychosomatic' (Weil 1983, pp.67–8).

This is a very challenging notion. It suggests that we need to find a way to make our treatments psychosomatic – which I take to mean that in the session we need to find a way to engage the patient's psyche in the work. Few of us have any training in this, and even if we did, our work is very different from that of a psychoanalyst. When we venture into this kind of thing with a patient, which we all have to do from time to time, we have no alternative but to use our intuition and learn from experience.

There is a tradition of classical Chinese medical case history where each practitioner finds a unique way of treating each patient. Two cases in the twelfth and thirteenth centuries are good examples: one where the treatment of a destructive and dangerous woman was to make her laugh; the other was of a patient who recovered from prolonged mourning by becoming angry. There are indeed many ways to get Qi to move. This is a truth not just in ancient practice and not just of Chinese medicine, for here is an account of the work of a late twentieth-century gastroenterologist:

> ...one of the most remarkable men I have known...told of his own experience with a serious illness when he was about thirty years old. His condition had commanded the attention of a number of doctors, but it had come to the point that they had more or less given up hope for him. For two weeks, he neither ate nor drank and nothing the doctors could do was helping. Finally they asked him if he would like to see a particular specialist...who was everywhere recognised as the top man in his field (what is now called gastroenterology)...
>
> [He said] 'I was very weak, but I remember...this little man coming right into my room without even looking at the charts, which were outside. He came in and sat by my bed and after a little while he just said (and here my friend laughed): "I think it would be a good idea to give you grapefruit juice." Then after a little while longer, he left.

And from then on I started to get better. And the fact is that this man was a healer...he conveyed something to me.' (Needleman 1985, p.163)

In the following quotation Ted Kaptchuk is referring to the ancient Chinese doctors whose cases I mentioned above, but what he says applies perfectly well to the previous story: 'Immediacy, intuition and even the outrageous are the currency of this type of encounter... Healing is beyond theories and therapeutics and includes the entire humanity of the patient and healer' (Kaptchuk 1997, pp.xvi–xvii).

So what is it that these doctors actually do? And how do they do it? And why does it always seem that their intervention is so minimal? The answers given by a wide variety of practitioners of long experience are expressed in different ways, but they all amount to much the same thing:

> When I asked Dr Schweitzer how he accounted for the fact that anyone could possibly expect to become well after having been treated by a witch doctor, he said I was asking him to divulge a secret that doctors have carried around with them ever since Hippocrates. 'But I'll tell you anyway,' he said, his face still illuminated by that half smile. 'The witch doctor succeeds for the same reason that all the rest of us succeed. Each patient carries his own doctor inside him. They come to us not knowing that truth. We are at our best when we give the doctor who resides within each patient a chance to go to work.' (Cousins 1979, pp. 68–9)

A cancer doctor with long experience concludes: 'I think that's what healing is – evoking the will to live' (Remen, cited in Moyers 1993, p.356).

Which leads on to a specific question:

> What is it that a doctor of any kind of medicine can do to initiate the will to live in somebody? Because obviously,

people cure themselves... I don't think it is a question of drugs or homeopathy...or acupuncture or anything of the sort. That's not the heart of the problem at all. (Needleman 1985, p.164)

Here is a master practitioner using a lovely analogy to explain how he does it:

Imagine a dancing party attended by a man who never dances... He always declines all invitations to participate saying he does not know how. One woman, however, likes the man sufficiently to persuade him to take the floor. Moving herself, she somehow manages to make him move too... At the end of the evening he finds he can follow her movements and steps more easily and can even avoid bumping into her feet... After going to a second party, he makes sufficient progress to shake his conviction that dancing is not for him... In saying that I work with people I mean that I am 'dancing' with them. (Feldenkrais, cited in Johnson 1995, p.143)

There is a clear relationship between this kind of dancing and the patient's will to live:

The point is that the good doctors of former times understood instinctively that a physically ill person often needs great external help in order to find internal force within himself. The effect...is that the patient discovers that what is being demanded of him is something he can do, that there is something in himself he can trust... That is to say, in illness all one's available psychic energy is being absorbed by bodily functions, and external help is often needed in order to free some of this energy for self-attention. Will in man is nothing if it is not free psychic energy. (Needleman 1985, p.76)

I am sure that some practitioners work consciously in this way, but much of what happens with a patient must be at least partly unconscious. When we have a clear diagnosis and treatment plan and when the patient improves from session to session then a powerful momentum builds up, which amplifies the precision of the practitioner's work and the patient's trust in it. By contrast, when we lose confidence in what we are doing, so does the patient, and the message that gets communicated from each to the other is something like: 'I am not at all sure about this.' You don't have to investigate the whole business of placebo effects to know that healing is much more likely in the first case than the second. And when we have those moments of intuitive knowing, those times when there is no doubt and everything is suddenly clear and simple, then the unconscious communication must be that all the tensions and confusions and uncertainties of illness are resolved. Even if it happens in a moment and is gone in a moment, it does open a window to the possibility of change and the prospect of health. Which may indeed be exactly what is needed to 'initiate the will to live'.

Unconscious communication also happens through the interaction of the energy fields of the patient and practitioner. In her research Valerie Hunt measured the energy fields of patients during treatment. She discovered that those fields were usually chaotic at the start but that they changed as the treatment went on and ended up like the more stable fields of their practitioners. This might be a clue as to how the great practitioners manage to do so much with so little – their energy itself is helping the patient to change. Whatever style of medicine they practise and whatever techniques they use, the real power of the treatment comes from the way their fields can have an effect on those of their patients and thereby restore them to proper functioning.

> We realised that a transaction between the two fields [i.e. that of the patient and that of the healer] was essential to hasten healing. When experienced healers had finished a...session the two fields...showed an identical pattern.

> Apparently, when healers sensed that identical pattern with the healee, they terminated the healing session... Electromedical researchers believe that each disease or functional disturbance has its own energy field which must be reversed before healing can take place. Probably illness is a disturbance first in the energy field and healing is the restoration of that field to health. (Hunt 1996, pp.28, 244)

This helps to explain a pretty common experience in the treatment room but one that I never understood before reading this. Imagine I have a treatment plan that involves needling five points bilaterally. After the third point I sense something has happened. I take the patient's pulses and they have improved enormously. Should I stick to the plan? Would the pulses get even better if I did? Usually my intuition tells me to stop. And it may be because I am sensing that the patient's energy field is no longer in the disturbed or erratic state it was but has come into alignment with my own.

Someone who has done no scientific research but has spent a lifetime studying doctors and what they do comes to a similar conclusion:

> I was not surprised to see that [Dr Kaufman] has in himself that specific quality that is shared by people who are what might be called 'natural healers'. I was not surprised to sense this quality as a distinct vibration... This energy...could express itself not only by a direct material action on the body and mind of his patients but could also to some extent select the thought associations in his own mind. This is intuition in its real meaning. (Needleman 1985, pp.173, 177)

Mutuality

There is one more routine assumption about illness and treatment that has to be challenged. Most of the time it doesn't matter much if we think of our treatment as something that only changes the patient, but that isn't entirely true when we base a treatment on intuition. Naturally we care about our patients, worry about them sometimes and learn from them in all sorts of ways, but what is involved here is a specific effect and has nothing to do with our normal concerns for their welfare.

When we do what we have been taught we are the inheritors of a great tradition, deserving of the utmost respect, and we are also following in the footsteps of our own teachers to whom we owe so much. It is how we all start to practise and how, most of the time, we continue to work. But when we begin to work intuitively there is a change. We certainly draw on the tradition and on our training, but there is an internal shift. Instead of being able to support our decisions by reference to the textbooks, to our college notes and to the teachings we have received at workshops and conferences – in other words justifying what we do by reference to an outside authority – we have to do so for ourselves. We have to provide our own validation.

And that has an effect on us, especially when we find ourselves acting on our intuition even though what it suggests seems implausible (everything pointed to tonifying Spleen, but I decided to needle Ki 3 and 25 instead), risky (I did a very big treatment on a patient who was weak from the stress of cancer tests) or upsetting (I said to a patient, 'I don't think I should treat you today; I think you need to see your doctor'). It feels quite naked.

> A commitment to awakening intuition is a commitment to truth. It implies a willingness to listen to the still small voice which you can recognise as being true, even when you don't

like what it says. It means a willingness to know yourself as you are, dropping pretences and disguises no matter how successful your particular act may be in terms of getting approval from others. (Vaughan 1979, p.176)

It is a big step to take, and not only in your practice. Once you start to do this in the treatment room then you will probably start to do it outside as well. After all, once you have been willing to 'know yourself as you are' at work it's hard to see how you can forget that knowledge when you are at home with your partner or your children. And then it gets built into your life. For, 'Each time you choose to take advantage of a new opportunity, trusting your intuitive sense of what is best for you, you are strengthening this habit, and the choices become easier and easier' (Vaughan 1979, p.41).

It helps you to relish your time with people as well. Marshall Rosenberg, the founder of the technique of non-violent communication, has found that it has led him to listen to people in a different way. I heard him say, 'I've learned that I enjoy human beings more if I don't hear what they think. I've learned to savour them much more by only hearing what's going on in their hearts.'

It also seems to be the way to avoid getting drained and exhausted by the work.

In my practice I see at least thirty people with cancer a week... People sometimes say to me, 'How do you stand this? How come you're not eaten alive?' But I'm not eaten alive at all. As a matter of fact, at the end of the week I feel fed and strengthened. Healing is natural. It's not something I do to you, but something that's mutual. (Remen, cited in Moyers 1993, pp.350–1)

In the end, it is all mutual. The practitioner's commitment to truth improves her own life and it evokes in at least some patients a willingness to see what is really going on, to acknowledge the true sources of their illnesses and perhaps to summon up the courage to make the changes that will start the process of healing.

CHAPTER 10

Conclusion

Whatever style of acupuncture is taught in the various colleges in the West what they all have in common is some kind of protocol for the work. My original training held that a proper diagnosis consisted of finding congruence among the following: the colour on the patient's face, the sound of his voice, the odour of the body and the emotional state that seemed to be awkward in some way and not flowing freely. And here is a statement of what might be called the TCM protocol:

> After making a diagnosis and identifying the pattern the next logical step is that of determining the principle of treatment to be adopted... The practitioner of Chinese Medicine will need to formulate a rational and coherent plan of action as to what should be treated first, what is primary and what is secondary in the patient's condition, what is the relative importance of the acute or chronic condition and what method of treatment should be used. (Maciocia 1989, p.311)

With both styles the procedure seems clear and straightforward, certainly by comparison with what is proposed in this book, but I think that is misleading. Either of them leaves plenty of room for doubt and disagreement, even among very experienced practitioners. Is this colour on the face really green or is it pale yellow? Is the patient's acid reflux primary or is it the dysmenorrhoea? Should Liver Qi Stagnation be dispersed first or the Spleen tonified? And I wonder how I would ever have time to get through all the stages of the second protocol, even if I mulled over each patient on my day's list before I started work.

There are deeper problems with it too. If your decision-making is based on collecting relevant information, how can you be sure what is relevant? Is it the patient's childhood experiences, the fact that he likes to go deep sea diving or an experience of a past life? And then how do you know when you have enough information? Presumably, you make a decision that what you have is adequate for the diagnosis, but how do you know that? I am sure there are areas of life in which it is possible to use the procedures of rationality, but in our work, where we have a very limited amount of time in which to make decisions about how to intervene in a system of staggering complexity, the truth is that we use our intuition all the time whether we know it or not. We act not when it is entirely rational to do so but when we sense that we have enough information, when we feel that the patient is getting tired of talking or when our body tells us that it's time to move; or even, to be honest, when we are running out of time.

And given that intuition seems to have been a well-known aspect of the work of skilled practitioners through the ages, it is curious that virtually no modern book on Chinese medicine even mentions it, and the few that do tend to explain it away.

> Among a certain segment of the population most interested in Chinese medicine in the West, intuition is valued above rationality. However, for me, intuition is merely the clarity of knowing something so well that one does not need to consciously and deliberately move through all the propositions of a syllogism. For me, the difference between rationality and intuition is merely speed and, in

my experience, training oneself to think clearly and logically
is the quickest and surest path to insight. (Flaws 1994, p.4)

In other words, intuition is alright as long as it is really only
following the standard protocol. I don't think this accords with
our everyday experience of intuition and it certainly seems to
be a rather modern Western view. The Chinese see it differently,
and in a way that may be more appropriate to the practice of
acupuncture.

This is best exemplified by the *I Ching* or *Book of Changes*,
which dates from before Confucius and which lies at the
foundation of Chinese thought. If you consult the book in
order to help you with a decision then, briefly, you do as follows.
First you compose yourself with some sort of ritual in order to
acknowledge the seriousness of the task and you formulate a
question that you want answered. Then you throw either sticks
or coins a number of times, recording how they fall each time.
The pattern thus created will correspond to one of the sixty-
four hexagrams in the book, and if you look it up you will find
a text that points to an answer to your question.

There are many ways of describing this process, but it
is reasonable to see it as a way of evoking and enhancing the
power of intuition. For one thing, the ritualistic start ensures
that no decision based on the *I Ching* will be taken lightly, and
intuition arrives most reliably when space and time are made
for it. For another, the text is poetic and suggestive, so the
interpretation that springs to mind when the book is consulted
will be one that resonates with what you were thinking already,
but perhaps didn't realise you were thinking. This is a good way
of avoiding the common error of making what seems to be a
sensible decision, which you then proceed to undermine because
unconsciously you are not happy with it. And finally, the whole
business of consulting the oracle depends on the notion that

each human being is part of the whole, part of the way the world works and turns; so the pattern made by the sticks or coins is bound to have the quality of that person in interaction with his environment at that precise moment. Any decision made on that basis will, the argument goes, have a deeper congruence with life as it is being lived than mere logic. And given that each of the hexagrams contains a sophisticated view of the dynamic interactions of Yin and Yang, what we learn from it is likely to be especially relevant to acupuncture.

Jung used the *I Ching* and commented on it as follows:

> The irrational fullness of life has taught me never to discard anything, even when it goes against all our theories (so short-lived at best) or otherwise admits of no immediate explanation. It is of course disquieting, and one is not certain whether the compass is pointing true or not; but security, certitude, and peace do not lead to discoveries. It is the same with this Chinese mode of divination. (Jung 1989, p.xxxiv)

I do love his acknowledgement of 'the irrational fullness of life'. For surely it is salutary to appreciate both the limitations of what we in the West think of as the strength and accuracy of rational thought and also to appreciate that other ways of thinking have coherent justifications of their own.

> I have learnt to trust my intuition and I have learned to do it sooner. It's taken a long time to realise that it isn't so important that I understand intellectually what I am doing. More important is that I feel the validity of my action... 'I feel it intuitively' is heard by some as a weak and waffling response. I don't care. I'm not going to resist actions based on my intuition just because I can't justify them. I don't find my judgmental faculty nearly as wise as my intuitive one. (Dass and Bush 1992, p.105)

Mastery

I recently asked one of the best-known and most-respected practitioners whether or not she worked intuitively and she replied: 'I don't just ask for help from my intuition, I demand it.' It made me think that mastery in acupuncture, as in other walks of life, comes from a combination of years of learning and experience and a willingness to call on intuition.

> I believe that the artist is someone more than usually blessed with a co-operative unconscious or sub-conscious, more than usually able to effect things with the help of instincts and intuitions of which he or she is not necessarily conscious. Like the great athlete, the great artist is at once highly trained and highly instinctual. (Ricks 2011, p.7)

These days we tend to use the language of the unconscious to talk about ideas, motivations and decisions that appear to arise without trace. Other times and other cultures use different language. The chakra system of India, for example, proposes that energy is focused at seven locations along the centre line of the body, and that each chakra enables a particular kind of awareness. The sixth chakra, located on the brow, just a bit higher than between the medial ends of the eyebrows and often called the third eye, provides unusual vision of remarkable clarity. Essentially, once the third eye is opened, then what is perceived is what cannot be seen with the other two eyes.

> Because the physical sense of sight is outward directed, it is constrained to the duality of observer and observed. Intuition, on the other hand, is an inner directed vision, a direct knowing in which knower and known are somehow engaged or even united. In Chinese medicine this point ...*Yintang* is sometimes referred to as *unnamed* because by naming we re-create the very duality that the third eye transcends. (Greenwood 2004, pp.161–2, italics in original)

In some Buddhist traditions a similar clarity of vision is thought to come from the heart, while a modern psychic healer reports: 'I found myself receiving information about the source of a client's illness. This information seemed to be coming from what appeared to be an intelligence higher than myself' (Brennan 1988, p.203). Whatever words are used to describe it, the experience is the same. It is reliance on a different source of knowledge, one that is available to everyone but only used by a few. That is because it only comes consistently and reliably to those who have practised calling on its aid.

For those acupuncturists who do so, there is no distinction between all the knowledge of Chinese medicine that they have accumulated over the years and the insight that comes in a momentary flash of intuition. It is not that logic entails one treatment while an unpredictable and wayward inner voice urges another. There is a congruence between learned knowledge and tacit knowledge, between the conscious and the unconscious, between the rational and the intuitive, between head and heart – there are many ways of expressing the dichotomy – which is the mark of a master practitioner. Many years ago I had the privilege of watching one of them at work and I was astonished by what I saw. Talking with each patient he seemed to have all the time in the world, but he saw more than twice as many people in a day as I do now. Then, once he started to needle, he moved without hesitation; he was sure-footed, going steadily from one point location to another rather like a freestyle climber reaching handholds on bare rock. At the time I was dazzled by his insights; now I am more impressed by his efficiency. When you know what to do, rather than having an idea what to do, then there is no need to mull, reconsider, pause for thought, change your mind and so on. Everything points to the same conclusion. As so often, all this is summed up much more elegantly by Lao Tzu:

The Master doesn't talk, he acts.
When his work is done,
the people say, 'Amazing:
we did it, all by ourselves!'

(Lao Tzu 1988, No. 17)

You

Learning to use intuition in the treatment room can be seen as a form of professional development, an enhancement of your skills as a practitioner and an added way of serving the patients who come to you. But if you choose to give it time and attention then it will make a difference to you too. Any practice that you take seriously – prayer, meditation, learning a language, playing an instrument – changes the way you see things and the way you respond to the challenges of your own life. Each practice has its own character and typical effects, but in this case, 'A commitment to awakening intuition is a commitment to truth' (Vaughan 1979, p.176).

That is not necessarily always easy. Sometimes the truth is unpalatable, sometimes it seems to make impossible demands of you, and it always illuminates who you really are as opposed to who you think you are. Still, in the end, the decisions that spring from a commitment to truth tend to work best. Deciding where to practise, how much to charge your patients, what courses to go on, how to talk to a teenage son who is in trouble or confront a partner whose behaviour is upsetting you – with all of them you can exercise 'the muscles of your intuition' and be open to the truths it will reveal. For, 'Only intuition gives true psychological understanding both of oneself and others' (Assagioli 1965, p.220).

Decisions might then start to come more quickly and more easily, both in and out of the treatment room. You might then start to live out the teaching of the Dao De Ching, which speaks always of allowing rather than forcing, of yielding rather than controlling and of the wisdom of spontaneity. You might even find yourself working with 'the unthinkable ingenuity and creative power of a man's spontaneous and natural functioning' (Watts 1962, p.27).

And that might have the most delightful of consequences, for 'what the culture of Taoism...proposes is that one might become the kind of person who, without intending it, is a source of marvellous accidents' (Watts 1962, p.27).

References

Assagioli, R. (1965) *Psychosynthesis*. New York: Hobbs Dohrman.

Ballentine, R. (1999) *Radical Healing*. New York: Rider.

Birch, S. (1997) 'A Case of Post Partum Complications?' In H. MacPherson and T. Kaptchuk (eds) *Acupuncture in Practice*. London: Churchill Livingstone.

Blake, W. (1975) *The Marriage of Heaven and Hell*. Oxford: Oxford University Press (original work published 1790).

Brennan, B. A. (1988) *Hands of Light*. New York: Bantam Books.

Chopra, D. (1989) 'The Spell of Mortality.' In R. Carlson and B. Shield (eds) *Healers on Healing*. Los Angeles, CA: Jeremy P. Tarcher.

Cousins, N. (1979) *Anatomy of an Illness*. New York: Bantam Books.

Darby, M. (2003) 'Professor J. R. Worsley: a personal tribute.' *European Journal of Oriental Medicine 4*, 3, 34.

Dass, R. and Bush, M. (1992) *Compassion in Action*. London: Rider.

Dass, R. and Gorman, P. (1986) *How Can I Help?* London: Rider.

Denmei, S. (2003) *Finding Effective Acupuncture Points*. Seattle: Eastland Press.

Eliot, G. (2003) *Middlemarch*. London: Penguin (original work published 1871–2).

Flaws, B. (1994) *Sticking to the Point*. Boulder: Blue Poppy Press.

Flaws, B. (1997) 'Pregnancy, Nausea and Multiple Sclerosis.' In H. MacPherson and T. Kaptchuk (eds) *Acupuncture in Practice*. London: Churchill Livingstone.

Fulford, R. C. (1996) *Dr Fulford's Touch of Life*. New York: Pocket Books.

Garner, A. (2014) *The Bronze Age Man of Jodrell Bank*. London: BBC Radio 4, 21 May 2014.

Gladwell, M. (2005) *Blink*. London: Penguin.

Goldstein, J. (1976) *The Experience of Insight*. Santa Cruz: Unity Press.

Greenwood, M. (2004) *The Unbroken Field*. Victoria: Paradox Publishers.

Hanh, T. N. (1976) *The Miracle of Mindfulness*. Boston: Beacon Press.

Hicks, A., Hicks, J. and Mole, P. (2004) *Five Element Constitutional Acupuncture*. London: Churchill Livingstone.

Hsu, E. (1999) *The Transmission of Chinese Medicine*. Cambridge: Cambridge University Press.

Hunt, V. V. (1996) *Infinite Mind*. Malibu: Malibu Publishing.

Johnson, D. H. (ed.) (1995) *Bone, Breath and Gesture*. Berkeley: North Atlantic Books.

Juhan, D. (1987) *Job's Body: A Handbook for Bodywork*. Barrytown, NY: Station Hill.

Jung, C. G. (1971) *Psychological Types*. London: Routledge (original work published 1921).

Jung, C. G. (1985) *Modern Man in Search of a Soul*. London: Ark Paperback (original work published 1933).

Jung, C. G. (1989) 'Foreword.' In *I Ching or Book of Changes*. London: Penguin Arkana.

Kahneman, D. (2012) *Thinking Fast and Slow*. London: Penguin.

Kaptchuk, T. J. (1989) 'Healing as a Journey Together.' In R. Carlson and B. Shield (eds) *Healers on Healing*. Los Angeles, CA: Jeremy P. Tarcher.

Kaptchuk, T. J. (1997) 'Preface.' In H. MacPherson and T. J. Kaptchuk (eds) *Acupuncture in Practice*. London: Churchill Livingstone.

Kaptchuk, T. J. (2000) *The Web that has no Weaver*. Chicago: Contemporary Books.

Lao Tzu (1988) *Tao Te Ching* (trans S. Mitchell). London: HarperPerennial (original work published in antiquity).

Maciocia, G. (1989) *The Foundations of Chinese Medicine*. Edinburgh: Churchill Livingstone.

MacPherson, H. (1997) 'Introduction.' In H. MacPherson and T. J. Kaptchuk (eds) *Acupuncture in Practice*. London: Churchill Livingstone.

Miller, J. (1978) *The Body in Question*. London: Jonathan Cape.

Milner, M. (1986) *A Life of One's Own*. London: Virago.

Moyers, B. (ed.) (1993) *Healing and the Mind*. London: Thorsons.

Mukherjee, S. (2011) *The Emperor of all Maladies*. London: Fourth Estate.

Myers, D. G. (2002) *Intuition*. New Haven: Yale University Press.

Needleman, J. (1992) *The Way of the Physician*. London: Arkana (original work published 1985).

Newby, E. (1975) *Love and War in the Apennines*. London: Penguin.

Ni, M. (trans) (1995) *The Yellow Emperor's Classic of Medicine*. Boston: Shambhala.

Oschman, J. L. (2000) *Energy Medicine: The Scientific Basis*. London: Churchill Livingstone.

Pert, C. (1997) *Molecules of Emotion*. New York: Scribner.

Polanyi, M. (1958) *Personal Knowledge: Towards a Critical Philosophy.* Chicago: University of Chicago Press.

Remen, R. N. (1989) 'The Search for Healing.' In R. Carlson and B. Shield (eds) *Healers on Healing.* Los Angeles, CA: Jeremy P. Tarcher.

Ricks, C. (2011) *Bob Dylan's Visions of Sin.* Edinburgh: Canongate.

Rolf, I. (1977) *Rolfing: The Integration of Human Structures.* New York: Harper & Row.

Rolf, I. (1978) *Ida Rolf Talks.* New York: Harper & Row.

Salk, J. (1983) *Anatomy of Reality.* New York: Columbia University Press.

Scheid, V. (1997) 'Ockham's Razor and a Case of Ankylosing Spondylitis.' In H. MacPherson and T. Kaptchuk (eds) *Acupuncture in Practice.* London: Churchill Livingstone.

Schultz, M. L. (1999) *Awakening Intuition.* London: Bantam Books.

Seem, M. (1997) 'A Crushing Pain in the Chest.' In H. MacPherson and T. Kaptchuk (eds) *Acupuncture in Practice.* London: Churchill Livingstone.

Sennett, R. (2009) *The Craftsman.* London: Penguin.

Shealey, C. N. and Myss, C. M. (1988) *The Creation of Health.* Walpole: Stillpoint.

Siegel, B. S. (1986) *Love, Medicine and Miracles.* New York: HarperPerennial.

Simon, H. A. (1992) 'What is an "explanation" of behavior?' *Psychological Science 3*, 3, 150–61.

Smith, R. (2014) *Barbara Hepworth Exhibition Guide.* Kendal: Abbot Hall.

Solfrin, J. (1989) 'The Healing Relationship.' In R. Carlson and B. Shield (eds) *Healers on Healing.* Los Angeles, CA: Jeremy P. Tarcher.

Updike, J. (1990) *Self Consciousness: Memoirs.* London: Penguin (original work published 1989).

Upledger, J. E. (1989) 'Self Discovery and Self Healing.' In R. Carlson and B. Shield (eds) *Healers on Healing.* Los Angeles, CA: Jeremy P. Tarcher.

Upledger, J. E. (1997) *Your Inner Physician and You.* Berkeley: North Atlantic Books.

Vaughan, F. E. (1979) *Awakening Intuition.* New York: Anchor Books.

Veith, I. (trans) (2002) *The Yellow Emperor's Classic of Internal Medicine.* Berkeley: University of California Press (original work published 1949).

Watts, A. (1962) *The Way of Zen.* London: Penguin Books (original work published 1957).

Watts, A. (1992) *Tao: The Watercourse Way.* London: Arkana (original work published 1975).

Weil, A. (1983) *Health and Healing.* Boston: Houghton Mifflin.

Weil, A. (2008) *Spontaneous Healing.* London: Sphere.

Wilbur, R. (2004) 'Walking to Sleep.' In *Poems of Sleep and Dreams.* New York: Alfred A. Knopf (original work published 1967).